YOU CAN
BE FIT!

A simple

guide to

understanding

fitness and

nutrition

D1307481

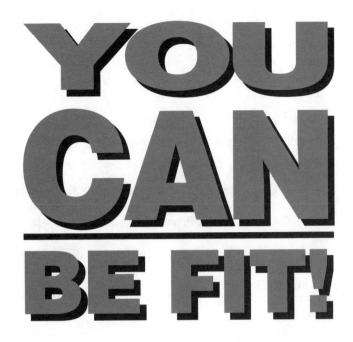

YOU CAN BE FIT!

A simple
guide to
understanding
fitness and
nutrition

Steven M. Horwitz, D.C.

Illustration and Design
Greg Morrill

The intent of the author is only to offer information of a general nature to you in your quest for physical fitness and good heath. Consult your doctor before beginning any fitness/nutrition program. In the event you use any of the information in this book for yourself, the author and the publisher assume no responsibility for your actions.

Contents

Foreword

I first met Dr. Steven Horwitz at the National College of Chiropractic in 1986. I was teaching a course in Chiropractic adjusting and I needed a subject whose problem was an injury to the shoulder. Dr. Horwitz volunteered and I proceeded to fix his shoulder with techniques that brought forth cries of anguish from his fellow students. I was greatly impressed by this young man's desire to learn everything that would be of value to a doctor interested in treating athletes. He demonstrated a keen mind and a real desire to help all people.

It has been a delight and pleasure that Dr. Horwitz and I have become good friends and work together at athletic meets where the welfare of the athlete is paramount and quickly achieved.

I recommend "You Can Be Fit!" for the outlook is not only based on experience but also first hand knowledge of maintaining good health, body conditioning and mental awareness. The reader can only benefit by being exposed to this health direction.

Fondly,
Jack Kahn D.C.

– Consultant to
  LA Raiders and
  Denver Broncos

– Co-attending chiropractor
  for the Mobile I
  Invitational Track and
  Field Championships

– Attending physician for
  the NCAA Division II
  Diving Finals

– Chiropractor to many
  Olympic and professional
  athletes

Acknowledgements

This book was inspired by my patients. I want to thank the many patients who were kind enough to read the manuscript in its many stages. They gave me valuable feedback on what information to include, how to organize it and how to make it easier to read and understand.

Thank you to Steven Seater, Executive Director of the Foundation for Chiropractic Education and Research, for encouraging me to write this book. I appreciate this wonderful opportunity.

Thank you to DeAnna Beck of the Foundation for Chiropractic Education and Research for her energy, time, patience and experience. It was a pleasure to work with her.

Dr. Peyton Davis, my nutrition professor at the National College of Chiropractic, contributed his valuable time and knowledge of nutrition to help me present the nutrition information in the book accurately. He also helped in referencing the material. Thank you for all your help and support.

Thank you to Dr. Beverly Teter for her expertise in nutrition and her review of the nutrition chapter of the manuscript.

Thank you to Drs. Phil Santiago, Bob Hazel, Robin Hunter, Blaze Toto, Karen Polichene, Alan Rousso and Mike Foggia for taking their time to review the manuscript and make suggestions.

Thank you to Dr. Tom McGovern, a good friend and colleague. I appreciate all of his help.

Thank you to Dr. Don Sebolt for reviewing the manuscript in its infancy. His many comments and suggestions helped make this an accurate and informative book.

Thank you to Pat Connolly and Laura Remaly for taking the time to help me improve the accuracy and quality of this book.

Thank you to Rich Schulman for all his help in putting this book together.

Thank you to my brother, Robert, without whose computer help I would be lost.

Thank you to my friends Robert Incorvaia for getting me started in weightlifting, to Koji Morihiro for my first and only weightlifting belt and to Drs. Neil Fried and Victor Poletajev for developing my weightlifting skills.

Thank you to my parents for always being there for me.

Introduction

You __Can__ Be Fit! Yes, even *you* can do it. Today is an exciting day for you as it is the beginning of your journey to a more fit and healthy you. Whether you are an accomplished exerciser or just a beginner, you will gain insight from this book.

This book began as a patient education tool. My patients constantly ask me questions about fitness and nutrition. I wanted to give them a single source of information on both topics. I scoured the book stores but was unable to find one book that covered these topics thoroughly yet concisely. I wrote a handout which, over the course of 5 years, grew into this book.

Regarding fitness education, I have often heard the phrase "If you are going to talk the talk, you must walk the walk." This book has not been written by a gym-rat or movie star turned fitness expert. It has not been written by a scientist, researcher or doctor who has never exercised. I am a chiropractor who started doing push-ups at age 14 because I saw boxer Ron Lyle do thousands of push-ups in his prison cell to stay in shape. I played competitive sports in high school and college. At Cornell University I took up running and ran two marathons (26.2 miles). Then I began to weight train. In chiropractic school I competed in powerlifting and bodybuilding, winning my class in the 1986 AAU Collegiate Mr. America Bodybuilding Championships. I continued my fitness education by becoming a Certified Chiropractic Sports Physician, a Strength and Conditioning Specialist and a Certified Personal Fitness Trainer.

I tell you this because I want you to know that I understand fitness from the athlete, fitness trainer and doctor points of view. My goal is for you to get started safely and correctly in your fitness/nutrition program and then continue it for the rest of your life. I want you to enjoy your journey to a fitter and healthier you.

Read this book in its entirety first. Don't worry about the specifics, just get a general idea of what's involved in getting started. Decide whether starting a fitness/nutrition program is for you, then read each chapter, one at a time, to learn exactly what to do.

Now, turn the page and get started!!!

YOU CAN BE FIT!

A simple guide to understanding fitness and nutrition

The recent boom in fitness and health consciousness has spawned a plethora of videos, books, TV shows and articles on exercise programs put together and touted by everyone from doctors, movie stars, TV personalities and jocks, to just about anyone who can get the media's attention. Thus, we have some very good and some very poor advice floating around. What follows are guidelines on how to start and stay with a safe, enjoyable, fitness/nutrition program. Listed below are what I call the Ten Commandments of Fitness and Exercise.

1. Goal Setting

2. Physical Examination

3. Consistency

4. Slow Start

5. Warm Up/Cool Down

6. Aerobic Exercise

7. Strength Training

8. Flexibility

9. Listening To Your Body

10. Nutrition

1
Goal Setting

Jane Fonda, dressed in tights and smiling, cries, "Make it burn," as she moves energetically. Arnold Schwarzenegger, his massive muscles glistening, says that he only does 20 sets for his chest. Joe Montana floats back and fires a 60 yard perfect strike to his receiver. STOP! Do not compare yourself to these folks! They have trained many hours a day for years to look and perform the way they do. Be realistic, don't be too ambitious at first.

What is the reason for beginning a fitness/nutrition program? Do you want to lose weight, develop a svelte physique, feel more relaxed, enhance your performance in a specific sport, have more energy or become more muscular? The number 1 reason for exercising, reported by 2 surveys - the Miller Lite Report on Sports and the American Health Survey on Fitness [1] - in which more than 50% of the respondents agreed, is to improve health. Setting a specific goal is a must to make your program a complete success. Define reachable goals for yourself. Set an ultimate goal with a time table for its completion. Then set interim goals so that, along the way, you are able to monitor your progress. Enjoy your journey!!!

2
Physical Examination

The American College of Sports Medicine has developed the following guidelines for beginning an exercise program: "Apparently healthy individuals can begin **moderate** (intensities of 40%-60% VO2 Max) exercise programs (such as walking or increasing usual daily activities) without the need for exercise testing or medical examination as long as the exercise program begins and proceeds gradually, and as long as the individual is alert to the development of unusual signs or symptoms." Apparently healthy men over 40, women over 50 and those who have at least two major coronary risk factors should consult a doctor and have a maximal exercise stress test. The major coronary risk factors are a history of high blood pressure, an elevated total cholesterol level (greater than 240 mg/dl), a family history of heart disease before age 55, diabetes mellitus or cigarette smoking.[2]

Stress Test

A maximal exercise test or "stress" test is done to aid in the diagnosis of heart disease. It is based on the premise that partial blockage of the coronary arteries (the arteries which supply the heart with blood) cannot be diagnosed simply by listening with a stethoscope or taking a resting electrocardiogram.[3] Exercise forces the heart to pump more blood than at rest and "stresses" the heart, enabling the cardiologist to determine if there are any obstructions or blockages. This test is performed by walking on a motorized treadmill or pedaling a stationary bike at increased elevation or resistance while having your blood pressure, heart rate, perceived exertion and electrocardiogram monitored.

Common sense dictates that even if you are not a man over 40 or a woman over 50 and do not have any of the aforementioned risk factors, you should inform your doctor that you have decided to pursue a fitness/nutrition program. You may say, "My doctor doesn't know anything about exercise," and you may be right, but he/she should know about your present state of health and whether or not you have any of the risk factors listed above (you should know as well).

3

Consistency

In America we have witnessed a fitness revolution that began in the 1980s. Pollster George Gallop surveyed this trend and called it the most important social phenomenon he had observed in a lifetime of assessing American attitudes. Up to 50% of adults shed their work clothes for athletic garb on any given day. Yet fewer than 20% of adults get enough exercise to have a positive impact on cardiovascular health and 40% of adults remain entirely sedentary.[4]

"Part of the problem is that people do not stay with exercise programs," says author James Rippe, M.D. "Drop-out rates 50% or higher within six months to a year are commonly reported." In his book *The Sports Performance Factors*, written with William Southmayd, M.D., Dr. Rippe continues, "Most people don't understand that the major benefit of exercise is the result of a lifelong consistent exercise program. Studies have shown that college or even Olympic athletes who stop exercising once their competitive careers are over quickly revert to the same risk of developing heart disease as if they had never exercised at all. Of course, you get some short-term benefits from starting an exercise program, but the most important benefits - decreasing the likelihood of heart disease, maintaining musculoskeletal strength and endurance, slowing bone density loss - belong to individuals who participate in lifelong consistent exercise programs." [5]

Establish a routine. Pick specific days of the week, a specific time of day, and a specific amount of time you can devote to your exercise program. Make it part of your everyday routine and then, **STICK TO IT!**

4
Slow Start

You wake up in the morning. You lift your head up in an effort to get out of bed and nothing happens. You try again and an explosion of pain engulfs your body as if you have been pummeled with a baseball bat. Were you a weekend warrior who played too many sets of tennis, played touch football for the first time since college, spent three hours lifting weights or rode that bike 20 miles after removing the cobwebs? You barely make it through the day and swear you will never exercise again, ever!

One of the reasons people do not continue an exercise program is that they overexert themselves at the beginning. They must then take time off due to pain or injury and ultimately lose the motivation to continue. This occurs often in aerobics classes where the number of injuries has skyrocketed over the past few years. **The highest rates of injury often occur at the beginning of an exercise program, so START SLOWLY!** You cannot make up for years of not exercising in a few weeks.

Clothing

Before you start your exercise program you need the proper clothing. Shorts or sweat pants, a t-shirt or sweat shirt and quality athletic shoes are a must. Find a sturdy, cushioned athletic shoe (cross training shoes work well) that will support your foot properly and is made to fit your activity. Do not perform weightlifting or aerobics in running shoes - they do not provide lateral (side to side) support so you are more susceptible to spraining your ankles.

Where Will I Train?

You have two options for where to train - at home or at a fitness center. Training at home means purchasing the necessary equipment. Having this equipment in your home enables you to exercise at your convenience no matter what the time of day or what the weather conditions are like outside. A fitness center relieves you of the need to purchase equipment, but it needs to be conveniently located.

Home Training

What is the necessary equipment? That's up to you, but you need to do aerobic, strength and flexibility exercises to have a complete fitness program. You can start with no equipment and try walking, calisthenics or following an exercise video (get an exercise mat if you perform floor exercises). Or you can go for broke and buy a treadmill, exercise bike, stair climber, rower, ski machine, free weights and a multi-station weight machine. For starters, I suggest 2 pairs of light dumbbells, a bench, and 1 piece of aerobic equipment (whatever you enjoy most). If you exercise at home, someone should be in the house while you workout. A training partner would be ideal. You must have a spotter if you use free weights. (See Appendix A: **How to Choose Home Equipment**).

Fitness Center Training

If you decide to work out at a fitness center, here are a few tips. There are three types of center - the hardcore weightlifting type, the health club (private or corporate) and the "medically" supervised fitness center. All come with different price tags, equipment and amenities; however, the following applies to all of them. Look for a club near your home; if it is not convenient you may never go. Consider joining with a friend as this can be a great source of encouragement to both of you. Check out the facilities at the time of day you expect to use them.

Questions To Ask

1. Is a new member given proper instruction on how to use the equipment? Is this instruction individualized for the member's needs and supervised by a qualified instructor?

2. Is adequate staff available in the exercise areas?

3. Is the equipment you need available?

4. Will there be lines for machines when you decide to go?

5. Is the equipment in good working order and serviced regularly?

6. Does the facility have adequate parking?

7. Does the facility have a first aid kit and ice available at all times?

8. If aerobic classes are given - are the instructors certified and are the floors properly padded?

9. Is there a water fountain in the exercise area? Is it clean?

10. Are child care facilities available? Are they clean?

11. Are the premises and locker rooms clean? Are lockers provided?

12. Are staff members CPR certified?

13. For how long is the facility bonded? Bonding requires the center, by law, to refund money to its members if it goes out of business. Example: If a club is bonded for 3 months and you join for 1 year and the club goes under, you will only get 3 months of dues back. Be wary of long term memberships and do not be rushed into signing.

There is no standardized certification needed to work in these facilities. Presently, there are many organizations that offer some type of fitness certification. The major organizations and their certifications are:

1. IDEA (International Association of Fitness Professionals) - In 1986 IDEA formed ACE (American Council on Exercise) to oversee certification programs. ACE offers certifications for Aerobic Instructors and Personal Trainers.

2. ACSM (American College of Sports Medicine) - They offer the following certifications: Exercise Specialist, Health Fitness Director, Health Fitness Instructor, Exercise Program Director, Exercise Leader and Exercise Test Technologist.

3. NSCA (National Strength and Conditioning Association) - Their certification is the Strength and Conditioning Specialist. Many professional and college strength coaches have this certification.

4. NASM (National Academy of Sports Medicine) - Their certification is called Personal Fitness Trainer.

5. AAAI/ISMA (American Aerobic Association International / International Sports Medicine Association). They offer the following certifications: Primary Aerobics, Advanced Aerobics, Step Aerobics, Personal Fitness Trainer, Weight Training Consultant, Nutritional Consultant and Fitness Expert.

6. AFAA (Aerobics and Fitness Association of America) - They offer a National Primary Certification that covers basic exercise standards and guidelines.

Some medically supervised fitness centers have medical doctors, chiropractors, physical therapists or athletic trainers on staff. Ideally, staff members should have some sort of health background.

Fitness Assessment

If you have decided to join a fitness center and their "trainer" is going to put you through your initial workout, do NOT let this be the **"let's see what you can do"** workout. If you feel like you are being pushed too hard (you feel dizzy, faint, experience pain or shortness of breath), **STOP!** You have the wrong trainer! The first workout should be a **"let me show you how to use the equipment"** workout. Some centers even put you through a fitness assessment before you begin your program. It usually consists of:

1. Height, weight, blood pressure, heart rate and health history

2. Body fat measurement - usually done with skinfold calipers

3. Cardiovascular endurance test (sub-maximal stress test) - you pedal a bike or step up and down off a block while your heart rate is monitored

4. A flexibility test (a sit and reach measurement)

5. A muscular endurance test (number of sit-ups you can do in a minute)

6. A strength test such as a bench press or push-ups

This type of analysis is used to determine your level of fitness when you begin and can be used as a comparison later.

Personal Trainers

For those of you who wish to start with a personal trainer, here are some things to consider:

1. Certification and Education: Some of the certifications are: a) Certified Personal Fitness Trainer by the National Academy of Sports Medicine; b) Personal Fitness Trainer by the American Council on Exercise; c) Fitness Instructor by the American College of Sports Medicine; and d) Strength and Conditioning Specialist by the National Strength and Conditioning Association.

Education should be a minimum of a Bachelors degree in either physical education, exercise science or exercise physiology.

2. All trainers should be CPR certified.

3. Experience - the more the better. Ask for references.

4. Fees - they begin at $25 per hour.

5. Do you go to the trainer or will the trainer come to you or your facility?

6. Enthusiasm - will this person get you motivated?

7. Define your goals for the trainer. Be wary of any trainer who fosters your dependence on him/her.

8. Your trainer should not be selling you nutritional supplements. Be wary of nutritional advice - check with a qualified nutritionist - an M.A., Ph.D. or R.D. (Registered Dietitian).

9. Your trainer is **not** your doctor and should **not** be treating your injuries. If you hurt, see a health care professional. (For more on injuries see Chapter 9: **Listen To Your Body**).

5

Warm-Up And Cool-Down

You wouldn't start your car, shift into drive, and step on the gas without warming up the engine first. Yet many people dive headfirst into a vigorous exercise routine without giving their body the same warm-up opportunity. Warming up and cooling down are necessary parts of an exercise program and are often forgotten or ignored when you are intent on packing a lot of exercise into a short time.

Warm-up

Warm-up is a term used to describe a variety of activities performed to prepare the body and mind for physical exertion. Warming-up is exactly as it sounds - elevating your body temperature one or two degrees above normal.[6] As a result, muscles and tendons become more lubricated and elastic allowing for more efficient contraction. The primary reasons athletes give for warming-up are performance enhancement and injury prevention.

The length of the warm-up depends on the type of activity involved, the level of intensity of the activity, and the level of fitness of the participant. For any activity, a general warm-up is necessary. This should last 5-15 minutes and may include walking, jogging or (stationary) biking with little resistance. If you are out of shape or new to a fitness program, walk or ride a stationary bike. If you run, start your run at a slow pace and gradually build speed over a 5-15 minute period. Elite athletes spend long periods of time warming-up. For example, the 100 meter dash takes about 10 seconds to run but sprinters will spend about **1 hour** warming-up before they race.

How will you know when you are warmed-up? When you break into a light sweat, you are ready to go. A warm-up should be task-specific as well. For instance, if you are going to lift weights, each body part you exercise should get its own warm-up. That means that if you are going to do bench presses, do your first set at a very light weight, 10-15 times. Then, **gradually** move up in weight. If you are going to play tennis, perform your general warm-up first and then volley for 10-15 minutes before you begin to play hard.

NOTE: Stretching is only part of warming-up and should be done **after** you break the light sweat from performing the aforementioned activities. (More about stretching is contained in Chapter 8: **Flexibility.**)

Cooling-Down

Cooling-down is best described by Bryant Stamford, Ph.D., in the journal *Physician and Sports Medicine.* "The cool-down is not as widely practiced as the warm-up but is no less important. Mild exercise enhances the disappearance of lactate from the blood which is thought to aid recovery. Cool-down is emphasized for swimmers and track athletes for recovery between events, but for other athletes it is ignored. Casual athletes, in particular, tend to ignore the importance of cool-down exercise. After a run, many individuals leave the track and immediately jump into their cars. Blood that has been diverted to the exercising muscles during exercise can pool in the legs when exercise stops abruptly. This reduces the return of blood to the heart which can shock the heart. [It is during this time when the heart is most susceptible to an arrythmia - an irregular heart rate or rhythm]. In addition, the muscles of the legs tend to tighten further, potentially causing pain, soreness, stiffness, and other problems. A cool-down exercise can be as simple as walking. Immediately following a run, brisk walking followed by walking at slower paces is recommended. Walking should continue until breathing returns to normal and the heart rate is near resting levels. At that point, perform a variety of slow, stretching exercises." [7]

6
Aerobic Exercise

"Aerobic" or cardiovascular endurance refers to the ability of the heart and lungs to supply oxygen and nutrients to working muscles. Increase this ability and you will be able to perform a task for progressively longer periods of time.

Applied to exercise, "aerobics" refers to any activity that raises the heart rate to a specific target range based on age and physical condition. Walking, bicycling, swimming, stepping, running, rowing and organized aerobic classes are just a few of the activities that can be aerobic and will help you become fit.

Fat Burning And Aerobic Exercise

Aerobic exercise burns fat. It will enable our bodies to become, as nutrition and fitness expert Covert Bailey says, "better butter burners." [8] When food enters your body it is broken down by enzymes. You can think of this as being done in 2 stages. In the first stage, these enzymes do not need oxygen to work; in the second stage they do need oxygen to work. The word aerobic means "with oxygen." It is the enzymes during this second stage-the aerobic stage-that break down fat to be used as energy by the body. As you become more fit, these oxygen-using enzymes grow larger and become even better fat burners.

When you exercise, your body uses both glucose (sugar in your blood, muscles and liver) and fat for energy. It is the relative amounts of each that you use that change as you become more fit. As you become more fit, you will be able to burn more fat and less sugar while you exercise.[9] You will start to peel off that excess fat and be able to exercise comfortably for longer periods of time.

An overfat person burns more sugar and less fat than a fit person. This is one reason overfat people tire easily. Even worse, since the amount of sugar in an overfat person's blood is low after exercise, this individual is more tempted to go out for burgers and beer because of hunger. Do not succumb to this temptation! Instead of burgers and beer, try skinless chicken and a baked potato (no butter or sour cream) and water or juice. (See Chapter 10: **Nutrition,** for more information).

Benefits Of Aerobic Exercise

The benefits of aerobic exercise are both physical and mental. Regular exercise will help reduce stress levels and give you a sense of well being, sometimes even euphoria. The physiological benefits are many - reducing your risk of heart disease, helping you lose weight and body fat, lowering your blood pressure, increasing your energy levels, decreasing your resting heart rate and increasing your maximum total body oxygen consumption (the combination of the blood pumped and the ability of the muscles to extract oxygen from the blood).[10] These benefits are only achieved and maintained if exercise is performed consistently and for your entire life. If you stop, these benefits will be lost quickly. Within a few short weeks, your aerobic fitness levels will drop if you stop exercising. Within a few months, it will be as if you never exercised at all.

Now, how do you get FIT? Follow the three general principles of any aerobic training program:

Frequency

Intensity

Time

Frequency is how many times a week you participate in your activity. Three times per week is sufficient for most individuals to achieve significant improvements in aerobic capacity. Increasing this to 4 or 5 times a week will cause further improvement. Training more than 5 days per week may increase your chances of injury.[11] (**Note:** Elite athletes' training programs are quite different, much more demanding, and quite specific to individual needs and requirements. Don't attempt to mimic their training regimens.)

Intensity means how hard you are working during your aerobic workout. Intensity can be assessed by monitoring your heart rate during exercise. This is done by taking your pulse in 1 of 2 areas: in the artery on the thumb side of the wrist (the radial pulse), or the artery in your neck just to the side of your wind pipe (the carotid pulse). Each artery has a left and right side. **Do not take your carotid pulse on both sides at the same time!** This will decrease blood flow to your brain! Practice finding your pulse. Your pulse rate is the number of times your heart beats in 60 seconds. Practice taking your pulse for at least 15 seconds (multiply the number of beats you count by 4), and preferably 30 seconds (multiply the number of beats you count by 2). The pulse is most accurate if taken for one minute. During aerobic classes, breaks are taken to monitor your pulse. These breaks are usually 6 seconds or 10 seconds long. For the 6 second break, multiply the number of beats you count by 10 (add a zero). For the 10 second break, multiply the number of beats you count by 6.

There are many ways to determine what is called your **target heart rate** - the heart rate you must maintain to achieve aerobic benefits. The easiest way to determine your proper exercise intensity is to use what is called the "talk test". If you can't keep a conversation with a partner while exercising you are pushing too hard - slow down! The technical term for this is rate of perceived exertion - it is graded on a scale of 6-20 with 6 being your body at rest and 20 being maximal exertion or exhaustion. You judge how hard you feel you are working. For most people the recommended range is 12-16.[12]

The more complex method of determining your heart rate requires figuring out your maximum predicted heart rate and your resting heart rate or pulse. Resting pulse is simply your pulse taken in the morning just before you get out of bed.

Maximum predicted heart rate is calculated by subtracting your age from 220.

Example: For a person age 40:   220 - 40 = 180 beats per minute

The maximum predicted heart rate is **180**. Please realize that the maximum predicted heart rate decreases with increasing age and varies considerably at all ages.

This method has 3 steps:

1. Compute your maximum predicted heart rate.

2. Multiply this number by 70%.

3. Multiply this number by 85%.

This gives you a range with a lower and upper number.[13]

Example: For a person age 40: 220 - 40 = 180 beats per minute

180 x 70% = 126 beats per minute

180 x 85% = 153 beats per minute

The target heart rate zone is 126 to 153. A 40 year old should keep his/her heart rate in this zone while exercising.

The following chart will enable you to easily figure out your target heart rate zone. Just find your age and move up to find the correct zone.

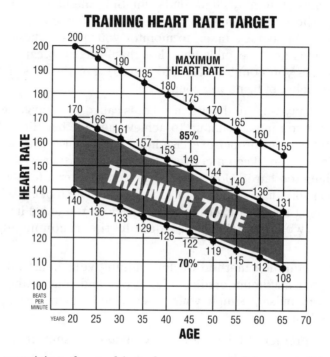

TRAINING HEART RATE TARGET

When exercising, the goal is to burn as much fat as possible for energy. Exercising in this target zone will allow you to do just that - it will make you a "better butter burner". If your heart beats too quickly you may burn too high a percentage of glucose (sugar in the blood) for energy (you may also overwork your heart to the point of injury). Therefore, you will not get the fat burning effects from your exercise. All you will do is end up feeling tired and hungry. If you exercise below the target zone you will not burn a significant amount of fat and your heart will not gain the desired aerobic benefits. People with heart disease or people taking medications that may affect the heart's response to exercise should ask their doctor for the best way to gauge exercise intensity.

Time - you must perform your exercise routine for **at least 20 minutes.** thirty minutes is quite sufficient, with 45 minutes to 1 hour a recommended maximum.[14] The health and fitness benefits taper off after 1 hour while the risk of over-use injuries increases dramatically. Each individual's rate of progression will vary. Some people may take only a few weeks to get up to 20-30 minutes of exercise, while for others it may take months. It is OK to start at 5 or 6 minutes and build from there. **TAKE YOUR TIME!**

Which Is The Best Exercise?

Walking is usually recommended for beginners but any exercise that meets the **FIT** criteria will do just fine. **The best exercise is the one you enjoy the most and will do consistently!**

Review

F	**Frequency:**	**3-5 Times Per Week**
I	**Intensity:**	**Talk test- you should be able to carry on a conversation while exercising**
T	**Time:**	**20 - 60 minutes**

(See Appendix B: **Aerobic Exercises: How to Perform Them Properly**).

7

Strength Training

Weights and Other Forms of Resistance Exercise

The National Strength and Conditioning Association defines strength training as "the use of progressive resistance methods to increase one's ability to exert or resist force." [15] Strength training often takes second fiddle to aerobics, but aerobic exercise is just for the heart. It is usually insufficient for developing muscular size and shape for that "hard body" look. Sometimes people are disappointed after doing aerobics for a few months when they don't see much change in the way they look. Resistance or strength training is what they need.

Let's clear up some misconceptions:

1. **Weight lifting is dangerous.** No, not if done with proper technique and progression.[16]

2. **If you stop, muscles will turn to fat.** No, physiologically that is impossible. Muscle cells are muscle cells and fat cells are fat cells. One cannot change into the other. Muscles will shrink and atrophy (lose size and tone)[17] if you stop exercising, and excess calories will be deposited as fat, giving the appearance of muscle turning to fat.

3. **Women will get big muscles.** First, most women build muscle size slower than men because they produce less of the hormone testosterone. Second, it takes years of vigorous training to build "big" muscles; it doesn't happen overnight.[18]

4. **You will get high blood pressure.** Strength training does not cause permanent high blood pressure although, during a lift your blood pressure does go up. Holding your breath while you lift weights does increase blood pressure dramatically, and is dangerous. Strength training may help lower your blood pressure over the long term.[19]

5. **You will become inflexible.** No, not if you include flexibility training as part of your overall exercise program. **As a matter of fact, if you do not exercise at all you will lose flexibility due to lack of use.**[20]

6. **Lifting weights lets me spot reduce a specific area of my body.** No, No, No, No! five thousand sit-ups every day will not give you the "washboard" stomach. First, to lose body fat from anywhere on the body, you must burn more calories than you consume. Second, when you lose fat, you lose it from the entire body, not just from one area. You lose it in proportions mostly dictated by genetic and metabolic factors. Third, exercises often done for spot reducing are relatively ineffective for burning fat and calories.[21] Cutting the excess fats from your diet, aerobic exercise **as well as** sit-ups will firm you up and flatten your stomach.

7. **I just want to "tone-up."** This term is usually used to describe a change from the flabby look to the "lean and mean" look. A toned muscle is simply a muscle that has been trained, is shapely and has that "hard as stone" look. What really takes place when you perform a proper exercise program and combine it with proper nutritional habits is a loss of body fat and an increase in muscle mass (size).[22] As was mentioned in misconception number 2, fat cells are fat cells and muscle cells are muscle cells. When you "tone-up", the fat cells get smaller and the muscle cells get bigger. Many people say, "I just want to tone-up; I don't want to look like a bodybuilder." When you strength train, you will build muscle. As long as you add aerobic exercise and eat properly, you will lose fat. The end result will be a lean but not heavily muscled look. You may notice some body parts get bigger more quickly than others but this is mostly due to genetics. If, for example, your legs are getting bigger than you wish, then just cut back on your leg training by decreasing the number of exercises and sets you perform for your legs.

Benefits Of Strength Training

The benefits of strength training are many: increased strength, improved muscle tone, enhanced athletic performance, increased bone, tendon and ligament strength, injury prevention and improved body image (self esteem).

It is being used in cardiac rehabilitation.[23] For women, one of the most significant benefits of weight training is that it reduces the risk of osteoporosis. Bones need regular resistance to stay strong. Weight training causes the muscles to pull on the bones which will then strengthen the bones.[24] This benefit does not occur to the same extent with aerobic exercise.

If your age is making you think twice about starting a weight training routine, think about this: The muscles of older people are just as responsive to weight training as those of younger people. Extensive research has shown great improvement in strength **in 80 and 90 year olds!** In one study, 80 and 90 year old people were trained with weights for 3-4 months. They were able to increase their strength 3-4 times over this period.[25] This has important consequences on the quality of living. It is muscular strength that is necessary to get in and out of a chair, walk up and down stairs, and to lift things. For some inspiration, take a look through the book *Growing Old is not for Sissies*, by Etta Clark.[26]

Strength Training Terminology

1. **Reps or repetitions.** This is how many times you move the weight up and down. For example, in the squat or deep knee bend, 1 rep would be lowering yourself down and raising back up 1 time.

2. **Sets.** This is a grouping of repetitions. For example, 3 sets of 10 reps means doing 10 reps, resting, doing 10 reps, resting, and doing 10 reps.

How Do I Start?

Strength training should be performed at least 2 times per week, leaving at least 48-72 hours between workouts. (**Note:** More advanced weight training may be performed more frequently and with less time between workouts. Discussion of this is beyond the scope of this book.) You must pick exercises for each of the body parts: legs (calves, front thigh, rear thigh), abdomen, back, chest, shoulders, and arms (biceps, triceps). Don't neglect any body parts - this will lead to imbalances in your body. Buy an anatomy book and learn the names of the muscles and what they do. This will be extremely helpful in learning how to do your exercise properly. (See Appendix C: **Functional Anatomy: Names of Muscles and What They Do,** for a brief overview.)

Proper Form

Proper form is critical when using free weights or machines. Proper form must be learned using the lightest weights possible before adding weight to your exercise. I suggest you use a personal trainer for your first 2-3 workouts. Having a qualified person watch and instruct you is invaluable. In this way, you will prevent injury and get the greatest possible benefits from your training.

How Much Weight Do I Use?

Start LIGHT! This means that when you first try an exercise, use the lightest weight possible. This will give you a baseline. Gradually add weight until you reach a weight with which you are able to do 10 reps **comfortably** and in **strict form.** You should not struggle to complete the 10th rep.

Once you have determined the correct weight to use, pick 1 or 2 different exercises per body part and start with 1 or 2 sets of 10 easy reps. Take 1 to 3 minutes between sets. If you are out of breath, just slow down. **Always use a light weight for 10 easy reps when performing the first set of a new exercise.**

Control The Weight

When you are performing a rep, you must **control the upward and downward movement of the weight.** Always lower the weight slowly and in a controlled manner. You may raise the weight quickly, but you must have full control and strict form. **You control the weight; never let it control you.** For example, in a bench press you slowly lower the weight to your chest (never bounce it on your chest) and then push up hard with control and strict form. This means that the only parts of your body that move are your arm and chest muscles. The rest of you remains stationary. **Never jerk the weights up and down!** A quick word about "negatives", i.e. having somebody help you lift the weight so you can slowly lower it: Don't do this in the beginning as it greatly increases your chance of injury and will make you quite sore!

Proper breathing is essential - breathe out when exerting yourself (as in the upward phase of a bench press) and breathe in when recovering. **DO NOT HOLD YOUR BREATH!** Make sure you have a spotter while weight lifting - someone who knows how to help if you get stuck.

Sample Exercises

Examples of exercises for each body part are:

1. **Chest -** Bench press, Incline bench press, Fly (Butterfly), Decline bench press

2. **Back -** Pull down (wide or narrow), Bent over row, Seated row, Dumbbell row, Pull-up, Chin-up

3. **Shoulders -** Shoulder press, Side raise, Front raise, Rear raise, Upright row, Shrug

4. **Arms -** Biceps: There are a multitude of curling exercises, Triceps: French Press, Push down, Kickback

5. **Midsection -** Abdominals: Crunches, Twisting crunches. Most abdominal exercises are done improperly and over-stress the lower back. Be careful when placing your arms behind your neck as there is a tendency to cheat and jerk the movement. You may want to cross your arms on your chest instead

6. **Legs -** Squat, Leg press, Lunge, Leg extension, Leg curl, Heel raise.

The order of your exercises should progress from the larger muscle groups (legs, back, chest) to the smaller ones (shoulders, arms, midsection).[27] The larger muscle group exercises require more mental concentration and use the most energy. (For more advanced weight training or sport specific weight training, performing the large muscle group exercises first may not be the most appropriate way to train - the specifics are beyond the scope of this book.)

Periodization

Progression in weight training should be done in a cyclical fashion. The technical term is periodization.[28] Training is divided into 4 to 8 week cycles. For example, whether you begin with 2 or 3 workouts per week, your first few weeks should include 1 or 2 sets of 10 reps per exercise. Work on perfecting your form. Over the next 4 to 8 weeks, you may wish to increase the number of sets to 3 per exercise. You may elect to add weight in small increments. The weight you choose should allow you to do 8 to 12 reps. For the first few months, stay in this range. After this time period, you may wish to exercise different muscles on different days.

To make further gains you must stress your muscles beyond the demands of your previous training. This is called the overload principle or progressive resistance training.[29] Milo of Croton demonstrated this principle in 300 B.C. by carrying a calf every day until it grew into a full-grown bull.

After you have been training for several months, vary your training by changing the number of sets and reps, the exercises you perform and the order of those exercises every 4 to 8 weeks. This is a very important point that is often overlooked.

Circuit Training

Another way to weight train is circuit training.[30] Many gyms have circuit training areas. A group of machines that exercise all of the body parts are used. You perform 1 set of 10-15 reps on each machine. You move from machine to machine with little rest (1-15 seconds) between machines. Circuit training is a good way to become fit. However, you will not increase your strength over the long term as much with circuit training as with free weight/machine training. Whether or not circuit training provides aerobic benefits is still controversial. Perform separate aerobic exercises to attain aerobic benefits.

Free Weights Versus Machines

For those of you out there who want to "tone up," stick with the machines as they are easier to use and are less likely to cause an injury. If you want the Arnold Schwarzenegger or Cory Everson look, free weights are the answer. This requires much more sophisticated lifting techniques and more practice at light weights. Probably the best way to train is to use a combination of free weights and machines.

If you wish to train at home all you really need is a few pairs of dumb-bells (2lb, 5lb, 10lb,) and a bench. (See Appendix D: **Sample Home Weight Training Program** and Appendix E: **Sample Weight Training Exercises for the Fitness Center.**)

Weight belts: The function of the weight belt is to prevent injury to the spinal discs, the shock absorbing pads between the spinal bones. The belt does this by spreading the force out around the midsection decreasing the pressure on the discs.[31] A proper belt is 4"-6" wide. Tighten it immediately before your lift and loosen it after the lift is completed. Wear a belt when using free weights. You may want to wear it on certain machines. Check with a qualified trainer. Do not let wearing a belt give you a false sense of security. Proper technique with the correct amount of weight for you is a must.

Review

1. Learn Proper Form; Control The Weight
2. Exercise All Body Parts
3. Start With 1-2 Sets Of 10 Reps
4. Start With A Weight With Which You Can Perform At Least 10 Reps
5. Do Not Hold Your Breath
6. Rest 48-72 Hours Between Workouts
7. Use A Spotter
8. Use A Weight Belt For Free Weights

8
Flexibility

Flexibility is a component of fitness that is either forgotten or taught improperly. In his book *Stretching,* author Bob Anderson says that stretching "helps you make the daily transition from inactivity to vigorous activity without undue strain." [32] When you are sedentary, your muscles react by shortening and atrophying. Flexibility exercises must be done in order to lengthen your muscles and tendons and allow you to regain the range of motion you once had. The benefits of stretching include: (1) reducing the risk of musculoskeletal injury, (2) enhancing performance, (3) promoting circulation and (4) relieving tension.

How To Stretch

Here are some guidelines on how to stretch properly. First, **do not bounce up and down!** This is a big **No, No!** It is like tugging back and forth on a brittle rubber band - it can break if forcefully over-extended. (You may see world class athletes doing this. For them it may be beneficial - do not mimic them!) Second, **warm up before you stretch.** A few minutes of walking or riding a bike will do the trick. The stretch itself is done by spending 10 to 30 seconds at the point where you just begin to feel a mild tension or pull and no more. The feeling of tension should subside as you hold your position - if it doesn't, back off. Breathe slowly and rhythmically, do not hold your breath. Repeat each stretch 2 to 4 times. More is not better - be careful not to overstretch as this may cause ligament, tendon or muscle injuries.

Take time to stretch after you workout. Stretch all of your muscle groups. It will take time to see a difference in your flexibility - give yourself a chance. The goal is not to become **Gumby**, it is to become more flexible than you are now. Your flexibility will differ at different times of the day. Usually, you are least flexible in the morning. As you move during the day, you begin to limber up. However, if you have been sitting all day, you will be less limber when you first get up than after you get moving. Most importantly, do not compare yourself with others in this or any other fitness activity. Some people are naturally very flexible and some are not.

(See Appendix F: **Sample Stretches**)

9
Listen To Your Body

It is amazing how many people who exercise do not understand the human body at all. As you begin your exercise program, pay attention to how your body feels before, during and after exercise. Learn what feels good and what feels uncomfortable. You will be able to make adjustments that will enhance your routine. Learn which muscles perform various movements. By learning to listen to your body, you will gain tremendous insight into what works for you. Keep a journal that describes how you feel during and after each workout. You may notice some interesting patterns.

Train, Don't Strain

Please do not pay attention to this "no pain, no gain" nonsense. Don't misunderstand - pushing yourself is OK and even necessary to make gains. However, pain is your body's way of warning you that something is wrong - pay attention and heed this warning! Replace "no pain, no gain" with **"TRAIN, DON'T STRAIN."** Many people play a sport in an attempt to get in shape. You must get in shape to play a sport! Start training weeks or months before the season opens, not the day before the first game, first ski trip or first tennis match.

R.I.C.E.

If you have pain while exercising, stop and remember **R.I.C.E.: Rest, Ice, Compression, Elevation.**[33] **Rest** - stop what you are doing and do not stress the area for at least 1 day. **Ice** the area as soon as possible for 20 minutes every 1 or 2 hours. Keep a thin towel between the ice bag and your skin to prevent frostbite. An alternative to an ice pack is ice massage. Freeze water in a Styrofoam cup. Hold the cup and massage the ice directly against the skin for about 5 minutes (till your skin turns numb). **Compression** - apply pressure to the injured area to decrease swelling. **Elevation** of the injured area above the level of the heart will help decrease swelling by allowing fluid to flow back toward the heart.

See a Certified Chiropractic Sports Physician, Sports Medicine M.D. or D.O.(Osteopathic physician)to get your problem evaluated and treated correctly if (1) pain persists for more than 1 week, (2) you can't move the injured area, or (3) you get an infection (look for spreading redness under the skin). You only have one body; take proper care of it.

R.E.S.T.

Before returning to exercise remember **R.E.S.T.: Resume Exercise below the Soreness Threshold.** It may be helpful to think about injuries in 4 stages:

Stage 1: You are able to exercise, but you have pain afterwards.

Stage 2: You are able to exercise, but you have pain during exercise. This pain does not affect the quality or quantity of your exercise, e.g. if you run, the pain does not affect how fast or far you run.

Stage 3: You have pain during exercise and it affects your performance, e.g. if you run, the pain slows you down or causes you to shorten your distance, or both.

Stage 4: You are unable to exercise at all due to pain.

When to return to your activity is best discussed with your doctor.

Muscle Soreness

You should NOT be sore after a workout! In the beginning, this may occur even if you are careful. Soreness after every workout does not mean your workouts are effective, it means you are doing damage to your muscles by not letting them recover properly.[34] Muscles grow by tearing down and building back up. The building up phase requires rest. Constant muscle soreness means you are not giving your body the time it needs to rebuild and grow. Adjust your routine to allow your muscles to properly recover. Ways to prevent muscle soreness include proper warm-up and cool-down, stretching and ice applied to the involved area immediately after exercise.

Do not underestimate the importance of resting. Recovery from your workouts is just as important as the workout itself. Many elite athletes, after being forced to rest due to injury or illness, return and perform at a higher level than before the injury. The symptoms of overtraining - fatigue, general body malaise, disinterest, sleeping difficulties, listlessness, sweating - are sure signs you need rest.[35] Either decrease the intensity of your workouts or just skip one.

10
Nutrition

A book on fitness would be incomplete without discussing nutrition. Exercise and proper nutritional habits go hand in hand. This section reviews basic nutrition as it applies to fitness. I hope it inspires you to do further reading on this important topic.

"THERE IS NO DIET NOW, AND THERE NEVER WILL BE A DIET, THAT CURES A WEIGHT PROBLEM. The reason for this is that diets don't attack the fundamental problem of the fat person. You see, most people think that losing weight is the basic problem.... Diets help people lose weight but losing weight is not the basic problem. The problem is - gaining weight! Fat people gain weight easily and quickly, so they soon have more fat than they have just lost," [36] says Covert Bailey, a leading authority on nutrition.

He adds, "We have developed such a mania for losing weight that we overlook what the lost weight may consist of. Suppose I were to call you on the telephone with the exciting news that the local supermarket was selling twelve pounds for only $1.29! Your reaction would be twelve pounds of what? Well, that is my reaction when someone tells me of a terrific diet which guarantees that you can lose twelve pounds in no time at all - twelve pounds of what?" [37]

Overfat

Most people are concerned with being overweight, but this term is obsolete. The proper term is **overfat.** Your body weight is made up of 2 major components: fat weight and lean body weight (muscle and bone). The relative amounts of each, expressed as a percentage of body fat, are what is important. People make the common error of regarding overweight and overfat as identical. Many sedentary people are excessively fat, but not overweight, while many athletes are overweight but not overfat. Take Arnold Schwarzenegger - at 6'1", he was 235 lbs. when he competed. Was he overfat? I don't think so! A 40 year old man may weigh the same as he did in college but may have not exercised since college, and he may think all is well. Surprise - he may have become overfat without a change in his body weight.

Fat can be divided into two types - subcutaneous (under the skin, the stuff we wish to lose) and intramuscular (like the marbling you see in a piece of meat at the supermarket). What has happened to the aforementioned 40 year old is that he has gained fat between the muscles but not much under the skin. He has become **fatter!!**

Unfortunately, most people get caught in the dieting trap. Growing evidence indicates that calorie restrictive diets (less than 800-1000 calories per day) cause the body to become very efficient at preserving energy - it slows down. "There is a dramatic and sustained reduction in resting metabolic rate. This causes the dieting to become progressively less effective. When the rewards of one's efforts are no longer apparent the dieter usually quits and reverts to previous eating habits." [38] When people regain weight after dieting (studies have shown that 50% will gain the lost weight back within two to three years), they tend to gain fat and lose muscle. Thus, their *new* body mass will have a higher percentage of bodyfat.[39]

If fat (weight) loss is your goal, reduce about 500 calories per day from your daily intake. Weight loss is a slow process; no more than 1 or 2 lbs should be lost per week.[40] An approximate **minimum** daily intake is 1500 calories for males and 1200 calories for females.[41]

Body Fat Measurements

If you lose weight too quickly you will be losing not only fat, but muscle as well. This is why it is wise to get a body fat measurement to be used as a baseline when beginning a fitness/nutrition program. There are many methods of body fat measuring: hydrostatic (underwater) weighing, skinfold (caliper) measurements, bioelectrical impedance and infrared. The most accurate method is hydrostatic weighing. The problem with this method is that few facilities have the necessary equipment. The skinfold (caliper) measurement is the most common method performed. This can be very accurate if done by an expert or grossly inaccurate if done by someone who is unskilled. If you have this done at a health club, ask to be tested by a qualified staff person. When you are retested make sure you have the same method performed by the same person under the same conditions. This will allow for a more accurate assessment of your improvement. Males should be no more than 18% body fat, females no more than 24% body fat.[42]

Energy = Calories

Energy is the body's first nutritional priority. The energy content of food is measured by a unit called a kilocalorie, which most of us call a calorie. Energy in food is supplied by fat, protein and carbohydrates. Protein and carbohydrates give 4 calories of energy per gram. Fat gives 9 calories of energy per gram.[43]

Due to this fact, it is not only the number of calories in your diet that is significant, but the composition of those calories as well. You need a balanced intake of carbohydrates, proteins, and fats. They can be taken from the 4 major food groups: (1)fruits and vegetables, (2) grains and legumes, (3) dairy products and (4) meats. About 60% of the total calories you eat should be from carbohydrates, 15% from protein and 25-30% from fat.[44] Even when you eat is important. Eat breakfast, a big lunch and a light dinner. Consume most of your day's calories before dinner.

Carbohydrates - These are the body's primary fuel source. There are two types, simple and complex. Complex carbohydrates get absorbed from the gut into the blood more slowly than simple carbohydrates. Good sources are fruits, pasta, rice, potatoes, breads and grains. They should account for 60-65% of your diet.[45] For serious athletes, this may be as high as 70%. Both your pre- and post-exercise meal should consist of mostly carbohydrates. Eat about 2 hours **before** and within 30-60 minutes **after** exercise to replenish the energy used by exercising. For those of you desiring weight (fat) loss, eat a small carbohydrate snack before and after exercise (e.g. a banana or bagel will work well) and stick to eating 3 well-balanced meals per day.

Protein - These are the building blocks of muscle, enzymes and some hormones. They are formed by units called amino acids (AA). There are over 20 different AAs and all must be present simultaneously for optimal growth and body functioning. There are 9 essential AAs - AAs that cannot be produced by the body so they have to be supplied by the diet. The remainder are nonessential AAs - AAs that can be produced by the body. Some foods are complete proteins (contain all the essentials AAs) and some are incomplete proteins (lack 1 or more of the essential AAs).[46]

Fish, chicken, beef, eggs and dairy products are complete proteins, whereas beans, lentils and vegetables are not. Vegetarians must combine foods properly to insure sufficient complete protein intake. The amino acids missing in one food must be found in another. Both of these foods must be eaten in order for your body to receive a complete protein source. Good sources of protein are fish, poultry, lean red meat, vegetables and legumes. They should account for about 15% of the total calories in your diet.

Fats - Almost all of what we read and hear about fats is negative and oversimplified. This has led to many misconceptions about fat. Fat is an essential energy source for the human body and is the major energy source for the heart. Without fat, the human body simply would not work. The main functions of fat are insulation, protection of organs, formation of essential fatty acids (fats that cannot be produced by the body so they have to be supplied by the diet), some hormone formation and energy storage. Fats are the most concentrated source of energy in the diet. They furnish twice the number of calories per gram than protein or carbohydrates. Fats should make up between 25% and 30% of your total daily caloric intake.[47]

There are desirable fats in fish oil, vegetable oil and olive oil. They may reduce the risk of heart disease.[48] The desirable fats found in fish oils are present in deep, cold water ocean fish like salmon and mackerel, not tuna. The breaded, deep-fat fried white fish from warm water, found in popular fish sandwiches, does not supply you with desirable fat!

There should be a balance of fats in one's diet, not a total ommission. The key is to lower the total fat intake. Avoid excess fat in dairy products, mayonnaise, sour cream, dressings, sauces, baked and fried goods. A food may have zero cholesterol but be high in fat content (e.g. peanut butter has zero cholesterol but it is 80% fat per serving). For those of you obsessive fat cutters, I'll leave you with a quote kept on the wall at a small town bakery: "More people die from worrying about calories [fat] than eating them."

Cholesterol - Cholesterol is needed to form male and female sex hormones, Vitamin D and cell membranes (especially in the heart). It is important for the brain and nervous system. Your body produces cholesterol in the liver. Outside sources of cholesterol come from animal fat only, not vegetable fat.

Much has been written about "good" and "bad" cholesterol or HDLs and LDLs. HDLs (good) and LDLs (bad) are particles which carry cholesterol (amongst other things) in the blood. HDL (high density lipoprotein) removes cholesterol from the tissues of the body and brings it to the liver. It has been shown to decrease the risk of heart disease. LDL (low density lipoprotein) carries cholesterol to the body tissues and, in excess, has been shown to increase the risk of heart disease.

The significance of HDLs and LDLs is their relationship to total cholesterol - the amount of cholesterol in the blood (expressed in milligrams percent- milligrams of cholesterol in 100 milliliters of blood). Total cholesterol should be 200 mg/dl or less. It is the ratio of total cholesterol to HDL and ratio of LDL to HDL, as well as the total blood cholesterol, that helps determine one's risk of heart disease (there are other factors as well).[49] When you have your cholesterol level checked, have your doctor explain these values and ratios and how they help determine your heart disease risk.

How To Read A Food Label

The Food and Drug Administration (FDA) states, "Grocery store aisles are on their way to becoming avenues to greater nutritional knowledge." By May, 1994, new food labels will be found on all packages of food. The new labels, says the FDA, "offer more complete, useful and accurate nutrition information than ever before." [50] Here is an example:

NUTRITION FACTS

Serving Size 1/2 cup (114g)
Servings per container 4

Amount Per Serving
Calories 260 Calories from Fat 120

	%Daily Value*
Total Fat 13g	**20%**
Saturated Fat 5g	**25%**
Cholesterol 30mg	**10%**
Sodium 660mg	**28%**
Total Carbohydrate 31g	**11%**
Dietary Fiber 0g	**0%**
Sugars 5g	
Protein 5g	

Vitamin A 4% Vitamin C 2% Calcium 15% Iron 4%
* Percents (%) of a Daily Value are based on a 2000 calorie diet. Your Daily Value may vary higher or lower depending on your calorie needs:

Nutrient		2000 calories	2500 calories
Total Fat	Less than	65g	80g
Sat Fat	Less than	20g	25g
Cholest.	Less than	300mg	300mg
Sodium	Less than	2400g	2400g
Total Carbohydrates		300g	375g
Fiber		25g	30g

1g Fat= 9 calories
1g Carbohydrates= 4 calories
1g Protein= 4 calories [51]

All food labels will have the new heading **Nutrition Facts**. Mandatory components of the label, in the order in which they must appear, are: total calories, calories from fat, total fat, saturated fat, cholesterol, sodium, total carbohydrate, dietary fiber - all in grams and % Daily Value. Also included are protein (grams), vitamin A, vitamin C, calcium and iron in % Daily Value. "Thiamin, riboflavin and niacin will no longer be required in nutrition labeling because deficiencies of each are no longer considered of public health significance." [52]

Daily Value: "A daily value intake of 2000 calories has been established as a reference. This value was chosen because it has the greatest public health benefit for the nation." [53] This does not mean that everyone in the U.S. should eat 2000 calories per day (that is why the 2500 calorie per day diet is included on the new label). Each person has different caloric needs. Elite athletes may eat 5000 to 7000 calories per day or more. This is what is necessary to sustain their performance levels. Discuss you caloric needs with your doctor and nutritional professional.

Please note that this new label does NOT give the PERCENT of the total calories per serving from fat. It tells you calories per serving - 260 - and calories from fat - 120. It does not tell you that 46% of the total calories are from fat. You must figure this percentage for yourself.

e.g. 120/260= .46 x 100 = 46%.

The information is somewhat misleading. The total number of grams of fat per serving is 13 grams. The **% Daily Value** listed is 20%. Read the paragraph noted by the asterisk. All of the **% Daily Value** information is for a 2000 calorie per day diet.

Dietary Dictionary: [54]

- **Free:** less than 5 calories; less than 0.5 grams of fat per serving; less than 0.5 grams of sugar; less than 5mg of sodium.

- **Low:** less than 140mg of sodium; less than 40 calories; 3 grams or less of fat per 100 grams of food.

- **High:** provides more than 20% of the amount recommended for daily eating, as in high fiber.

- **Reduced:** 1/3 the calories; 1/2 the sodium, fat, saturated fat or cholesterol.

- **Less:** 25% or less the sodium, calories, fat, saturated fat or cholesterol.

- **Light:** 1/3 fewer calories. Any other use of the term must specify that it is a reference to look, taste or smell, as in "light in color."

- **More:** at least 10% more of the nutrient, as in "more fiber," "more potassium."

- **Fresh:** raw food, never frozen, processed, or preserved.

- **Lean:** cooked meat or poultry with less than 10.5 grams of fat and less than 94.5mg of cholesterol per 100 grams.

- **Extra lean:** cooked meat or poultry with less than 4.9 grams of fat and less than 94.5 mg of cholesterol per 100 grams.

Vitamin and mineral supplements. It is important to realize that supplements are just that - additions to your diet that will balance any nutritional deficits. If you eat a balanced diet, you will receive all or almost all of the vitamins and minerals you will need without supplements. A multi-vitamin/mineral supplement with about 100% of the RDA (Recommended Daily Allowance) for each vitamin and mineral may be a good idea. However, if 1 tablet is good, 2 are not necessarily better. You will not only waste a great deal of money but may cause yourself more harm than good if you ingest megadoses. On the flip side, some research has shown that you may need as much as 3500 to 5000 calories per day to receive the trace minerals (i.e. selenium, chromium, molybdenum - no U.S. RDA has been established for these minerals as of the publishing of this book).[55] A trace mineral supplement may be a good idea. Please talk to your doctor or nutrition professional before embarking on a supplement program.

Do not forget the importance of water. It is the most important nutrient of all. You will only survive a maximum of 7 days without it. It makes up about 50-60% of the human body. The daily requirement is 8 8-ounce glasses per day (if you expend 2000 calories per day. If you expend more calories, you need more water.) [56] That means water - not coffee, not tea, not soda, not beer and not even juice. Thirst is not a good indicator of your need for water. Weigh yourself before and after exercise. You should not lose more than 2% of your body weight from exercise, so drink at regular intervals whether or not you are thirsty. Greater than a 5% loss of body weight can lead to serious injury and even death. Replace each pound of weight lost with one pint of water.

During intense exercise you may lose up to 1oz. of water per minute through sweat. The body can only distribute 1oz. per 3 or 4 minutes. Therefore, you must prehydrate - 16 oz. 30 minutes prior to exercise is a good guideline. Drink cool water (not ice water) as this is absorbed the most quickly.[57]

The easiest way to know if you have had enough to drink is to monitor your urine. Clear urine in significant amounts indicates adequate hydration. Dark-colored urine is concentrated with metabolic waste and means that you are dehydrated.

The Beginning

The beginning? You thought you just *finished* this book? You did! Now you must actively **begin** your fitness and nutrition program with the knowledge you have gained. As the people at *Nike* say, "Just Do It!" My mother used to quote an old saying. "Tomorrow, tomorrow, never today, say all lazy people."

Exercise and proper nutrition go hand in hand. All the programs, diets, etc., which emphasize just one or the other are incomplete. Put the two together and the quality of your life will increase dramatically. One of the greatest joys in my practice is to see a patient take this action and experience the wonderful benefits. Covert Bailey has said that if exercise could be made into a pill it would be the most often prescribed pill in the world.

Enjoy every day of your life and put some life into each day. I will leave you with the wise words of author and champion bodybuilder, Bill Pearl, "Physical health is seldom cherished until it is lost, and in the effort to regain it, we begin to realize what we wasted and threw away."

You CAN Be Fit!

APPENDIX A:
How to Choose Home Equipment

All equipment should include a manual and warranty. Service should be available if needed.

Checklist

1. Is the equipment sturdy? It should not shake when you use it.

2. Does the dealer deliver and assemble the equipment?

3. Are the gauges easily readable?

4. Can the equipment be adjusted to your height?

5. For Weight Equipment:

    a. Do the weights move smoothly?

    b. Is it easy to change the amount of weight you wish to use?

    c. Does the machine put you in the proper body positions while working the different muscle groups?

6. Is the equipment quiet?

7. Will the equipment fit in the space (including height) you have allotted?

APPENDIX B - Aerobic Exercises:
How to perform them properly

1. **Walking:** Purchase a quality pair of walking shoes. Keep proper posture - the ears should be over the shoulders and the shoulders should be centered over the hips. Keep a regular arm motion. Keep your arms down and do not clench your fists (this causes you to stiffen your posture). **Walking with hand weights** - this is not necessary and may cause injuries. If you use a treadmill, keep it level in the beginning as hill training is more advanced. On a treadmill, do not rely on the arm rails. Also, be careful when getting on and off.

2. **Stationary Bike:** Proper seat height - sit on the bike with the ball of your foot on the pedal - your knees should be slightly bent (15 degrees) at the bottom of the stroke. Some bikes have adjustable handles - keep your body as upright as possible. Begin your ride with easy resistance and gradually work your way up. Perform 60 to 90 revolutions (once around with the pedal) per minute. For those of you who find an upright bike too strenuous on your lower back, try a recumbent bike, it may provide more support.

3. **Step Machine:** Keep your body upright as in walking. Do not lean forward to rest your arms or hands on the rails, this places too much pressure on your back. Keep a loose grip on the arm rails. Putting too much pressure on the elbows can cause an irritation similar to tennis elbow. Leaning too heavily on the wrists can cause irritation and an injury like Carpal Tunnel Syndrome (nerve irritation at the wrist).

4. **Rowing Machine:** Maintain a steady, smooth motion. Do not curl your back when you move forward, bend at the waist. As you move backwards, pull with your arms, push with both of your legs and extend your back until you reach a position just past being upright. Using your legs is very important as there is a tendency to overuse the lower back muscles when performing this exercise. Do not jerk the handle bar. Do not jerk your neck.

   Note: Many of the aforementioned machines have different program and level settings. In the beginning, select the program that keeps your resistance steady. Begin at level one. Do not use the hill or interval training settings until you become more fit.

5. **Running:** Proper shoes are a must. Make sure you have about 1 thumb width of space between your big toe and the end of the shoe. Once you find a good pair of running shoes, buy 2 pairs and alternate with each workout. Be wary of always running on a hard surface as this can put excess stress on the joints. If you run on a track, reverse

directions each workout. Running on the same side of the road can also cause problems, similar to running in the same direction along the beach. Regularly running on the incline of a road can cause muscular and alignment problems in the lower extremities, pelvis and spine. To exaggerate, think of walking with one foot in the street and one foot on the sidewalk. Just imagine the imbalances this would cause over time. Try to run on a flat surface. Do not run in the middle of the road. Finally, if you run after sunset, wear a large, bright reflector!

6. **Outdoor Cycling:** It is important to have a properly fitted bicycle. A knowledgeable salesperson will properly fit you to your bike. Important points are stand-over clearance, saddle shape, saddle height, frame size and saddle to handlebar distance. Always wear a helmet!

7. **Cross Country Ski Machine:** Maintain an upright posture.

8. **Swimming:** Proper form is important. Review your stroke with a qualified instructor. Improper form can put excess wear and tear on your body, especially the shoulder area.

9. **Aerobics Videos:** Quality varies widely. Stick with a low impact or step program. Most of the recognizable names have good programs. Many videos have been medically reviewed. Check the labels. Clear an adequate space in front of the TV. Use an exercise mat. Wear the proper shoes. Monitor your heart rate. Do not compete with the instructor. Do not become dehydrated and remember that VCR's have pause and stop buttons.

10. **Aerobic Classes:** Do not perform high impact aerobics, especially as a beginner! Low impact and step aerobics are much safer. Make sure your instructor is properly certified. If you cannot keep up or you find a movement too difficult - STOP! Too many injuries occur when you compete with others. Go at your own pace.

For those of you who must carefully monitor your heart rate, purchase a pulse monitor. Purchase the type that has a lead that straps around your chest and sends an impulse to a watch you wear on your wrist. Certain pulse monitors will allow you to pre-program your target heart rate and will beep when you go above or below it. I suggest this for any of you who have heart problems or who are very out of shape. Consult your physician.

APPENDIX C - Functional Anatomy:
Names of muscles and what they do

Chest: **Pectoralis (Pec)** - These muscles push. They bring the arms from an arms out at side, parallel to floor position, to an arms directly in front of body, parallel to floor position.

Shoulders: **Deltoid (Delt)** - These muscles bring arms from arms at sides to arms overhead.

Back: **Latissmus Dorsi (Lat)** - These muscles pull. They allow the arms to pull in toward the body from an arms straight out position.

Legs: **Quadriceps (Quad)** - Front thigh- These muscles straighten out the knee from a bent position.

                Hamstrings (Ham) - Rear thigh- These muscles bend the knees.

                Calf- Gastrocnemius and Soleus - These muscles raise the heel. They allow you to stand on your toes.

Arms: **Biceps- Front arm** - These muscles bend the elbow. They are also used in pulling.

                Triceps- Rear arm - These muscles straighten the elbow. They are also used in pushing.

Abdominals: **Rectus Abdominus** - This muscle runs from the bottom ribs to the pubic bone. It brings these 2 areas closer together. If you perform a crunch, you bring your ribs toward your pubic bone while keeping your pubic bone stationary.

Lower Back: **Erector spinae** - These muscles parallel the spine on the left and right. These muscles straighten your spine from a bent forward position.

MAJOR MUSCLE GROUP

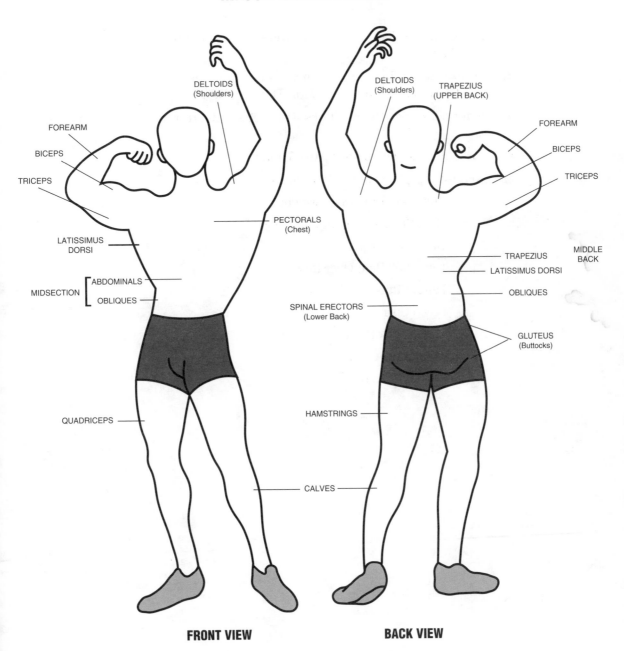

FRONT VIEW

BACK VIEW

DELTOIDS (Shoulders)

FOREARM

BICEPS

TRICEPS

LATISSIMUS DORSI

MIDSECTION — ABDOMINALS — OBLIQUES

PECTORALS (Chest)

QUADRICEPS

CALVES

DELTOIDS (Shoulders)

TRAPEZIUS (UPPER BACK)

FOREARM

BICEPS

TRICEPS

MIDDLE BACK

TRAPEZIUS

LATISSIMUS DORSI

OBLIQUES

SPINAL ERECTORS (Lower Back)

GLUTEUS (Buttocks)

HAMSTRINGS

APPENDIX D:
Sample Home Weight Training Program

1. Equipment needed: Dumbbells: Women 2lb. and 5lb.; Men 2lb., 5lb., 10lb. Weight bench.

2. Perform the following program 2 times per week with at least 48 hours between workouts, i.e. Mon/Thurs or Tues/Fri.

3. Perform 2 sets of 10 repetitions with a 60 second rest period between sets.

4. Workout length should be 30 to 45 minutes.

5. Exercises - perform in the following order:

    Lunge - start with no weight

    Heel Raise - start with no weight

    Bench Press

    Dumbbell Bent Over Row

    Lateral Raise

    Bicep Curl

    Tricep Kick Back

    Abdominal Crunch

    Back Extension

Suggested List Of Weight Training Exercises That You Can Perform At Home

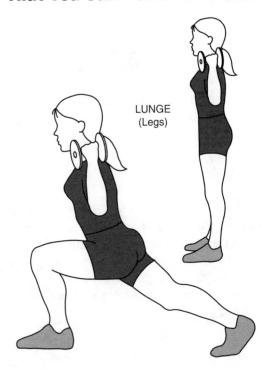

LUNGE
(Legs)

LEGS: Lunge - Stand with dumbbells in your hand, palms facing toward your body, feet together. While keeping your upper body straight, step forward on one leg. Lower slowly until your front thigh is parallel to the floor. Raise up slowly and breath out. Balance may be difficult so begin with a short stride and lengthen it as your balance and strength improve. Repeat 10 times for the left and 10 times for the right.

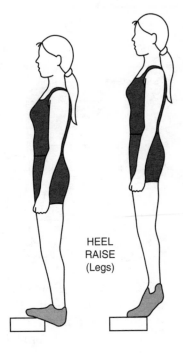

HEEL
RAISE
(Legs)

CALVES: Heel raise - Raise both heels simultaneously off the ground as high as you comfortably can. Slowly lower and repeat 10 times.

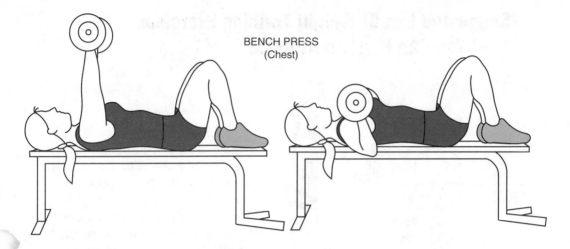

BENCH PRESS
(Chest)

CHEST: Dumbbell Bench Press - Lie on your back on a weight bench with a dumbbell in each hand. Keep your feet flat, either on the bench or on the floor. Start with your arms straight up in the air, palms facing your feet. While breathing in lower the weights slowly until the weights are along side your chest. Exhale while, in a controlled manner, you push up until your arms are straight. Keep your buttocks on the bench and your feet stationary. Repeat 10 times.

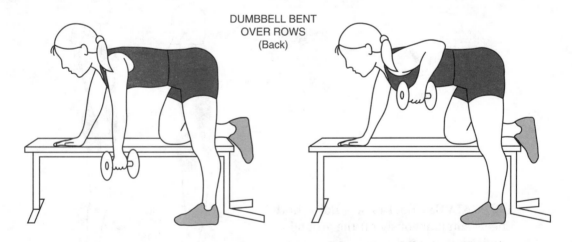

DUMBBELL BENT
OVER ROWS
(Back)

BACK: Bent Over Row - Place one hand and knee on a bench with your back flat and parallel to the floor. Grasp a dumbbell with your palm facing toward your body. Pull the dumbbell up to your chest while breathing out. Keep your back flat and parallel to the floor. Lower slowly until your arm is straight. Repeat 10 times with each arm.

SHOULDERS: Lateral (side) Raise - Stand or sit up straight and grasp dumbbells at your sides with your arms straight. Raise your arms to the side (like flapping wings) with your palms facing down. Keep your wrists straight and elbows slightly bent. As you exhale raise your arms until they are parallel to the floor. Lower slowly and repeat 10 times.

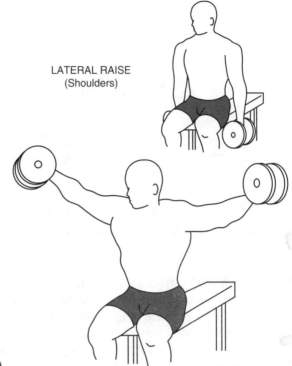

LATERAL RAISE
(Shoulders)

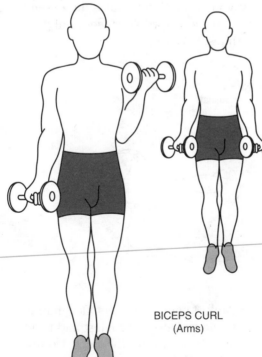

BICEPS CURL
(Arms)

ARMS: Biceps Curl - Stand straight with a dumbbell in each hand, palms forward. Keeping your elbows at your sides, slowly bend your elbows, bringing the weights up toward your shoulders. Slowly lower. Alternate arms and repeat 10 times.

TRICEPS KICK BACK
(Arms)

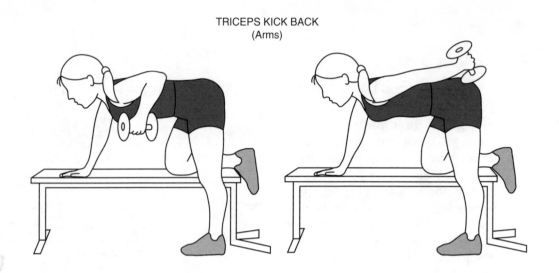

ARMS: Triceps Kick Back - Place one hand and knee on a bench, positioning yourself so your back is flat and parallel to the floor. Grasp a dumbbell with the other hand. Start with your arm (shoulder to elbow) along your side and bend your elbow to 90 degrees with the dumbbell hanging down, palm facing your body. Keeping your arm along your side, extend (straighten) your elbow moving the weight back toward your feet until your elbow locks. Slowly lower and repeat 10 times.

CRUNCH
(Midsection: Abdominal)

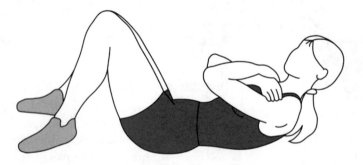

ABDOMEN: Crunch - Lie on your back, knees bent, feet flat, hands crossed over your chest to the opposite shoulder. Raise your chest and head while exhaling. Raise up until your shoulder blades are off the floor. Do not jerk or bend your neck. Keep your spine in line. Hold for 1 to 3 seconds, and breathe out while lowering. Repeat 10 times.

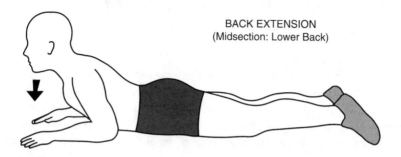

BACK EXTENSION
(Midsection: Lower Back)

LOWER BACK: Back Extension - Lie on your stomach, elbows under your chest, palms down. Raise your chest and head up until your elbows are at 90 degrees. Do not arch your head back and keep your spine in a straight line. Lower slowly and repeat 10 times.

APPENDIX E:
Sample Weight Training Exercises For
The Fitness Center

Four exercises per body part are given. These exercises are not the only ones you may perform. There are a multitude of exercises, both machine and free weight, for each body part. These are only a guide. Realize that certain fitness "experts" will have favorite exercises, but no one exercise should be etched in stone as the only one to do. As you become more experienced with weight training, incorporate a variety of exercises for each body part into your routine.

Have an instructor review how to use each of the machines and how to perform the free weight exercises you choose. Learn the proper body positioning and height adjustments for each machine. With free weights, learn the proper technique from the outset. You will prevent injury and progress more quickly this way. For all free weight exercises use a spotter. Never hold your breath. Breathe out when exerting force, i.e. when pushing up on a bench press or pulling down on the lat pull down exercise. Make sure you have the same amount of weight on each side of the bar. Grasp the bar or dumbbell with a thumb over the bar grip. Always move the weight in a slow, controlled manner. Never jerk the weights. In all lifting movements keep your head stationary. Again, make sure to pick at least one exercise per body part.

Sample Program

Start with a full body weight training program 2 or 3 days per week. Those of you who have never weight trained or are over 30 may want to start at 2 times per week. Make sure you wait 48 hours between workouts, i.e. Mon/Wed/Fri. Start with 2 sets of 10 repetitions with about 60 seconds rest between exercises. Workout length - 1 hour.

Perform the following exercises in the order given:

1. Leg Press

2. Leg Extension

3. Leg Curl

4. Chest Press

5. Pec Dec (Butterfly)

6. Back Pull Machine

7. Pull Over Machine

8. Shoulder Press

9. Lateral Raise

10. Biceps Curl

11. Triceps Extension

12. Abdominal Crunch

13. Lower Back Machine or Extension

Chest Exercise Guide

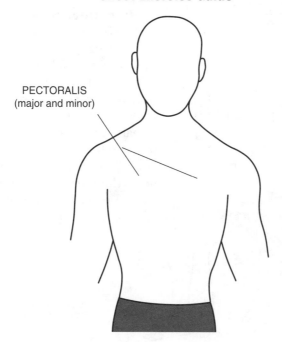

PECTORALIS
(major and minor)

MACHINE CHEST PRESS
(Chest: Pectoralis)

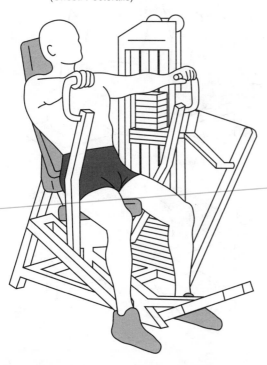

Machine Chest Press: You may be sitting up straight or lying on your back for this type of machine. Grip handles with thumb over grip. Push out foot plate to bring handles into starting position. Lift weight by pushing until your elbows are straight. Lower slowly. Do not jerk the weight. Do not hold your breath; breathe out when pushing.

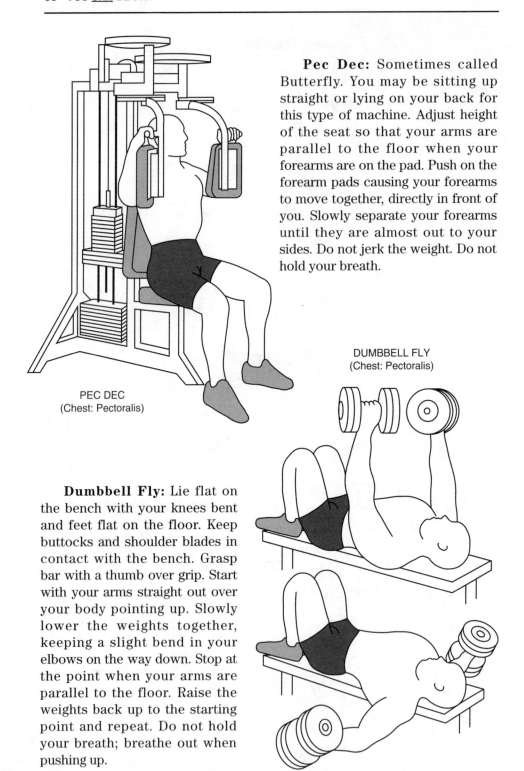

Pec Dec: Sometimes called Butterfly. You may be sitting up straight or lying on your back for this type of machine. Adjust height of the seat so that your arms are parallel to the floor when your forearms are on the pad. Push on the forearm pads causing your forearms to move together, directly in front of you. Slowly separate your forearms until they are almost out to your sides. Do not jerk the weight. Do not hold your breath.

PEC DEC
(Chest: Pectoralis)

DUMBBELL FLY
(Chest: Pectoralis)

Dumbbell Fly: Lie flat on the bench with your knees bent and feet flat on the floor. Keep buttocks and shoulder blades in contact with the bench. Grasp bar with a thumb over grip. Start with your arms straight out over your body pointing up. Slowly lower the weights together, keeping a slight bend in your elbows on the way down. Stop at the point when your arms are parallel to the floor. Raise the weights back up to the starting point and repeat. Do not hold your breath; breathe out when pushing up.

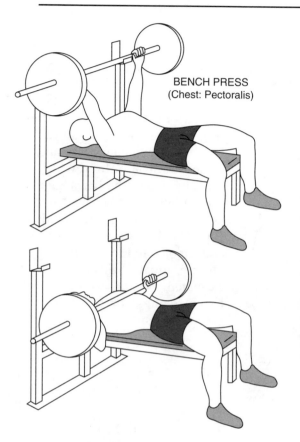

BENCH PRESS
(Chest: Pectoralis)

Bench Press: Lie flat on the bench with your knees bent and feet flat on the floor. Keep buttocks and shoulder blades in contact with the bench. Do not arch your back. Use a thumb over the bar grip. The width of your grip should be such that when the bar is fully lowered to your chest, your forearms are straight up and down (vertical). Lower the bar slowly to your chest, in line with your nipples. Do not bounce the bar on your chest. Raise the bar, pressing up and slightly backward so that at the completion of the lift, the bar is over your collar bone. Do not hold your breath; breathe out when pushing up.

Back Exercise Guide

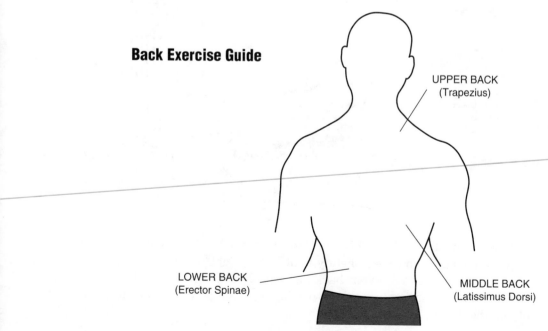

UPPER BACK
(Trapezius)

LOWER BACK
(Erector Spinae)

MIDDLE BACK
(Latissimus Dorsi)

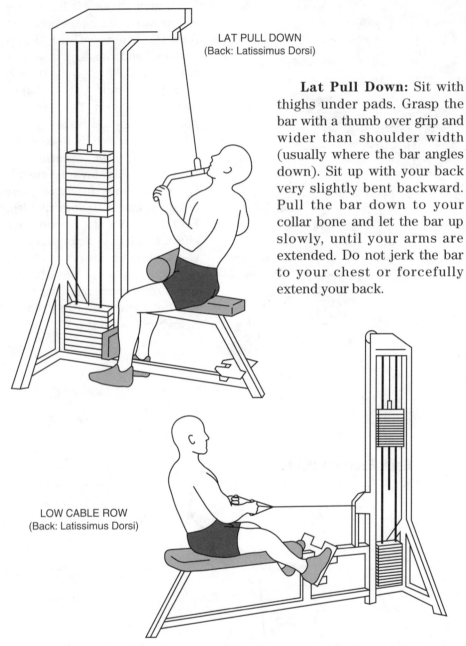

LAT PULL DOWN
(Back: Latissimus Dorsi)

Lat Pull Down: Sit with thighs under pads. Grasp the bar with a thumb over grip and wider than shoulder width (usually where the bar angles down). Sit up with your back very slightly bent backward. Pull the bar down to your collar bone and let the bar up slowly, until your arms are extended. Do not jerk the bar to your chest or forcefully extend your back.

LOW CABLE ROW
(Back: Latissimus Dorsi)

Low Cable Row: Place feet firmly on foot plates. Grasp handle and sit upright on seat. Keep knees slightly bent. Lift weight by pulling handle in, toward your torso. Extend your back just past 90 degrees. Lower the weight slowly, going forward no more than to a 45 degree angle with your torso. Do not jerk the weight. Do not hold your breath.

DUMBBELL BENT
OVER ROW
(Upper Back: Posterior Deltoid)

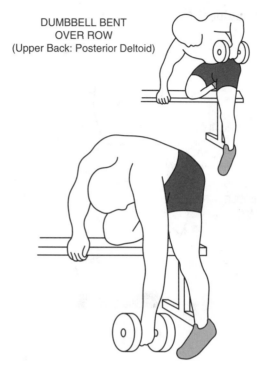

Dumbbell Bent Over Row:
Place one hand and knee on a
bench with your back flat and
parallel to the floor. Grasp a
dumbbell with your palm facing
toward your body. Pull the
dumbbell up to your chest while
breathing out. Keep your back
flat and parallel to the floor.
Lower slowly until your arm is
straight. Repeat with each arm.

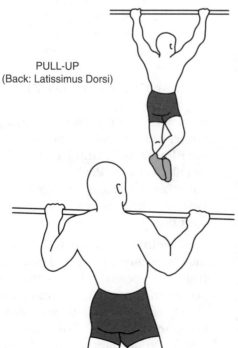

PULL-UP
(Back: Latissimus Dorsi)

Pull-up: Technically this
means your grip is palms away
from your body. A chin-up is
palms towards your body. Your
grip can be shoulder width or
wider. Pull your body up so your
chest almost touches the bar
and then slowly lower until your
elbows are almost straight.
There are some machines which
will help displace some of your
body weight with your feet, legs
or thighs resting on a pad. You
select how much weight you
wish to be displaced. This
allows you to do a pull-up with
less than your body weight. Do
not hold your breath.

Shoulders Exercise Guide

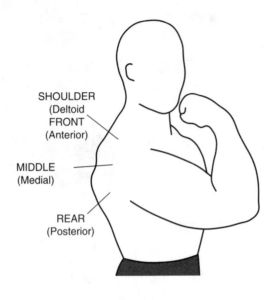

SHOULDER
(Deltoid
FRONT
(Anterior)

MIDDLE
(Medial)

REAR
(Posterior)

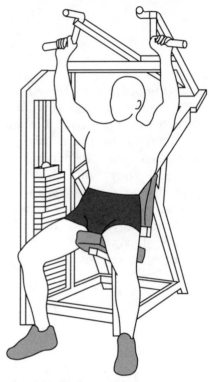

MACHINE SHOULDER PRESS
(Shoulders: Deltoids)

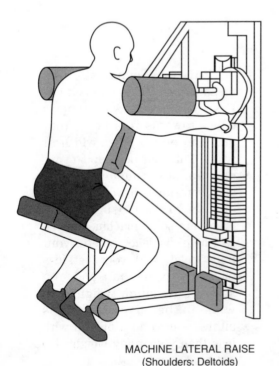

MACHINE LATERAL RAISE
(Shoulders: Deltoids)

Machine Shoulder Press: Adjust seat so that handles are level with your shoulders. Sit up straight and maintain contact with your lower back. Grip handles with thumb over grip. Push up until your elbows are straight. Slowly lower. Do not jerk the weight. Do not hold your breath.

Machine Lateral Raise: You may be seated facing into or away from the machine. Place outside of your arms against the pads and slowly raise them until your arms are parallel to the floor. Slowly lower. Do not jerk the weight. Do not hold your breath.

Dumbbell Shoulder Press: Sit with your lower back supported. Grip the dumbbells with thumbs over grip, palms facing away from your body. Start with the dumbbells at the level of your shoulders. Push upward until your arms are extended. Slowly lower to the starting position and repeat. Do not jerk the weight or arch your back. Do not hold your breath.

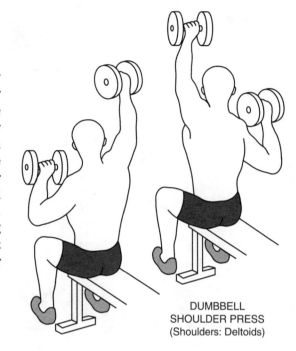

DUMBBELL
SHOULDER PRESS
(Shoulders: Deltoids)

Lateral (side) Raises: Stand or sit up straight and grasp dumbbells at your side with your arm staright Raise your arms to the side (like flapping wings) with your palms facing down. Keep your wrists straight and elbows slightly bent. Raise until your arms are parallel to the floor as you breathe out. Lower slowly and repeat 10 times.

LATERAL
(side)
RAISE
(Shoulders: Deltoids)

Leg Exercise Guide

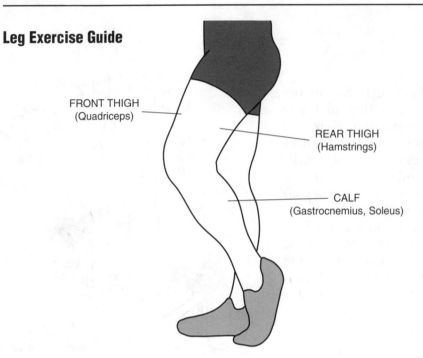

FRONT THIGH
(Quadriceps)

REAR THIGH
(Hamstrings)

CALF
(Gastrocnemius, Soleus)

Leg Press: Place feet on platform in desired position. Make sure knees are directly above the toes during the movement. If your toes point straight, your knees move straight. If your toes point out, your knees move out. Maintain contact of your back and shoulders with the pad. Lower the weight in a slow, controlled manner. Lift weight up by straightening the knees. Never jerk the weight up or drop down quickly. Do not hold your breath; breathe out when moving up.

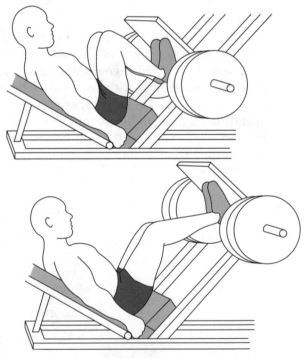

LEG PRESS
(Buttock/Thigh: Gluteal Muscles,
Quadriceps, Hamstrings)

Leg Extension: Adjust shin pad so that the pad comes in contact with your lower shin, just above your ankle. Align your knee with the axis of rotation by adjusting the seat back. The back of your knees should be snug against the seat. Lift the weight in a controlled manner. Do not swing or jerk the weight up. Lower slowly. Do not hold your breath; breathe out when straightening your knees.

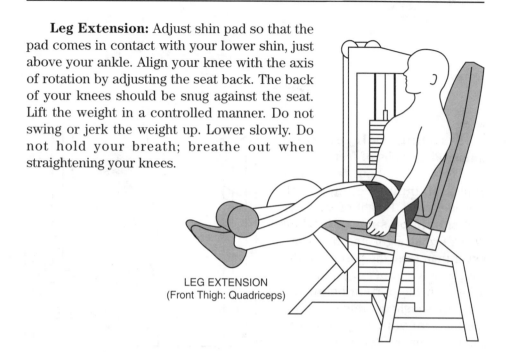

LEG EXTENSION
(Front Thigh: Quadriceps)

Leg Curl: Lie face down on the bench with your legs under roller pad, so pad is at back of your ankle. Keep your knees free of contact with bench pad. Grip handles lightly. Lift weight by curling heels up to buttocks in a controlled manner. Slowly lower the weight. Do not hold your breath; breathe out while bringing heels to buttock. There are two other common leg curl machines, one type is a seated curl, the other is a standing curl.

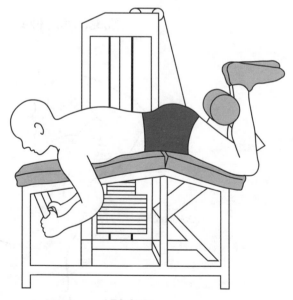

LEG CURL
(Rear Thigh: Hamstrings)

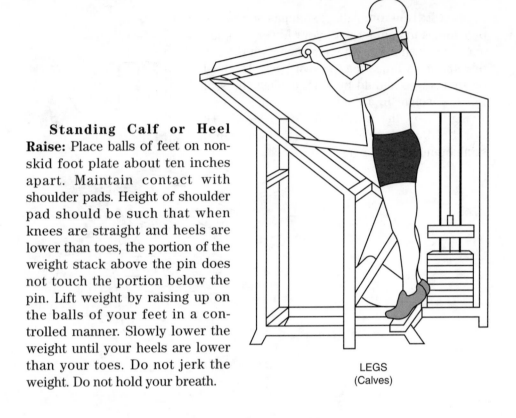

Standing Calf or Heel Raise: Place balls of feet on non-skid foot plate about ten inches apart. Maintain contact with shoulder pads. Height of shoulder pad should be such that when knees are straight and heels are lower than toes, the portion of the weight stack above the pin does not touch the portion below the pin. Lift weight by raising up on the balls of your feet in a controlled manner. Slowly lower the weight until your heels are lower than your toes. Do not jerk the weight. Do not hold your breath.

LEGS
(Calves)

Midsection Exercise Guide

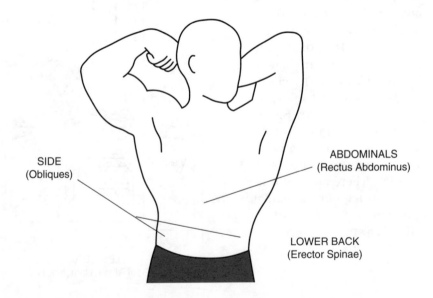

SIDE
(Obliques)

ABDOMINALS
(Rectus Abdominus)

LOWER BACK
(Erector Spinae)

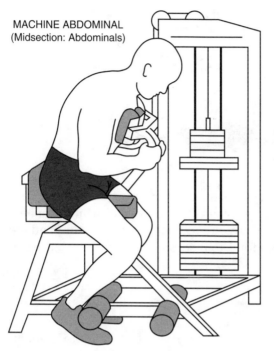

MACHINE ABDOMINAL
(Midsection: Abdominals)

Machine Abdominal: Adjust the seat position for proper axis of rotation (have the trainer help you). Slowly curl the pad forward for about 30 degrees of movement. It is not necessary to bend the torso completely forward. Return to the starting position slowly. Do not jerk the weight! Do not hold your breath; breathe out when curling forward.

Machine Back Extension: Adjust seat pad so that hips align with the axis of rotation (have the trainer help you). Slowly extend back until your body is straight. Slowly let weight forward until you have moved about 30 to 45 degrees. Do not go all the way forward or all the way backward. Never jerk the weight. Do not hold your breath.

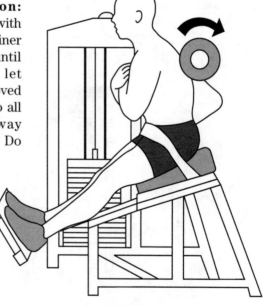

MACHINE BACK EXTENSTION
(Midsection: Erector Spinea)

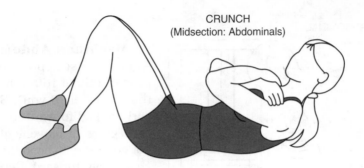

CRUNCH
(Midsection: Abdominals)

Crunch: Lie on your back, knees bent, feet flat, arms crossed on your chest to the opposite shoulder. Raise your chest and head while exhaling. Raise up until your shoulder blades are off the floor. Do not jerk or bend the neck. Keep the spine in line. Hold for 1 to 3 seconds, and breathe out while lowering.

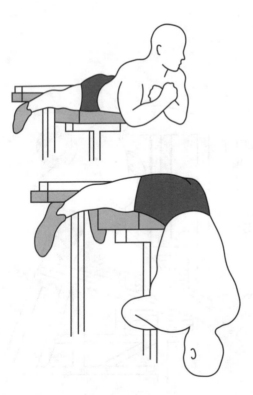

Back Extension: Commonly called a hyperextension. Start with your torso hanging off the pad at 90 degrees to your thighs. Uncurl your torso upward, until your torso is in line with your thighs. For some types of equipment this will mean your torso is parallel to the floor; for other types, your torso may be angled upward. The finishing position is when your torso is in a straight line with your thighs (like standing up straight). Lower your torso about 45 degrees and return. Perform this exercise as a reverse curl up and not just an up and down motion at the hips. Do not hold your breath.

BACK EXTENTION
(Midsection: Erector Spinea)

Arm Exercise Guide

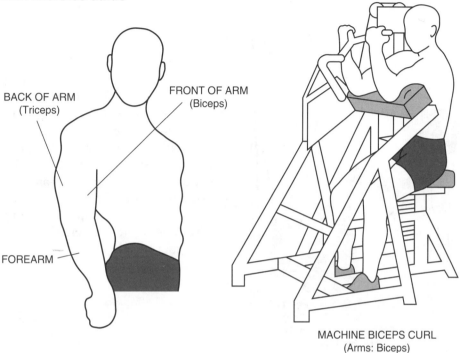

BACK OF ARM
(Triceps)

FRONT OF ARM
(Biceps)

FOREARM

MACHINE BICEPS CURL
(Arms: Biceps)

Machine Biceps Curl: Adjust the seat pad so that your elbows line up with the axis of rotation. Place chest against pad. Curl the weight all the way up and slowly lower until your elbows are almost straight. Never jerk the weight. Do not hold your breath.

Machine Triceps Press: This machine may be the exact reverse of the arm curl or you may be pushing two handles down toward the floor. Do not hold your breath.

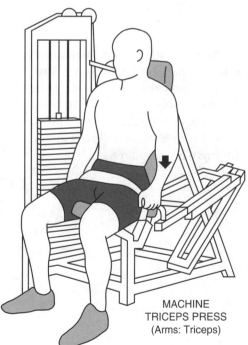

MACHINE
TRICEPS PRESS
(Arms: Triceps)

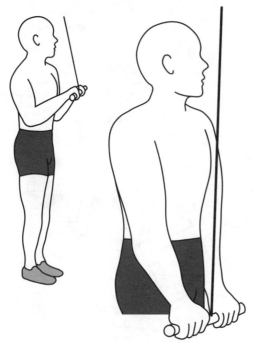

Triceps Push Down: Grip bar (straight bar or "V" bar) with thumb over grip, with hands about 6 inches apart. Start with the bar at chest level and your elbows at your sides. Keep your arms stationary and extend (straighten out) your elbows. Slowly return to the starting position. Do not lean your body over the bar when pushing down. Stand up straight throughout the exercise. Do not hold your breath.

TRICEPS PUSH DOWN
(Arms: Tricep)

Biceps Curl: Stand up straight, with a dumbbell in each hand, palms forward, keeping your elbows at your sides. Slowly bend your elbow, bringing the weight up toward your shoulder. Slowly lower. Alternate arms and repeat.

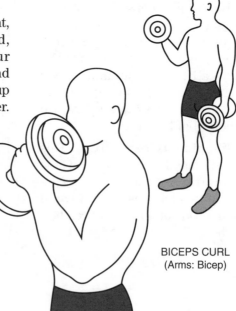

BICEPS CURL
(Arms: Bicep)

APPENDIX F:
Sample Stretching Routine

1. Be relaxed and warmed-up
2. Enter the stretch position slowly
3. The stretch should be comfortable
4. Hold for 10-30 seconds, relax, repeat
5. Breathe normally – do not hold your breath
6. Stop stretching if you have pain
7. DO NOT BOUNCE!!!

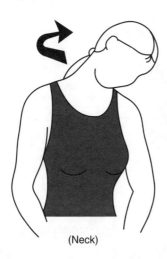

(Neck)

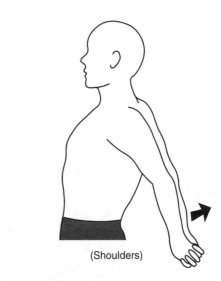

(Shoulders)

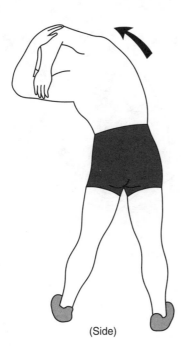

(Side)

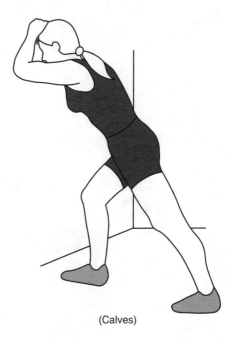

(Calves)

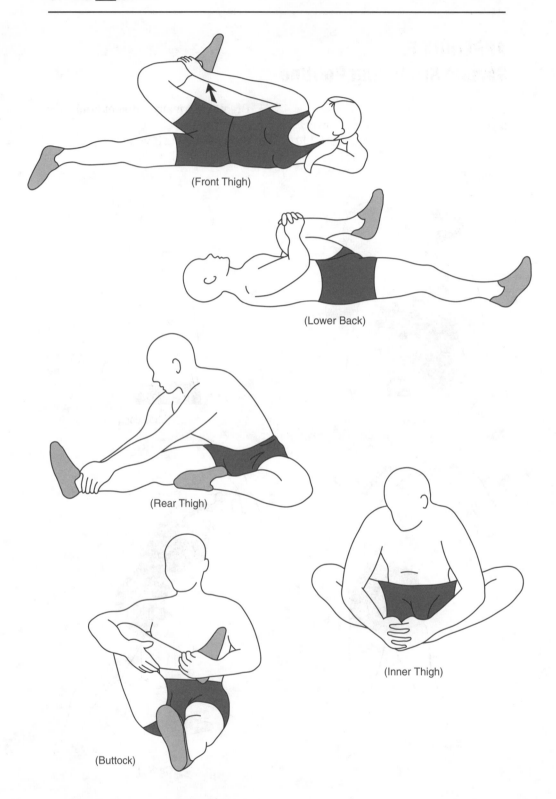

(Front Thigh)

(Lower Back)

(Rear Thigh)

(Buttock)

(Inner Thigh)

APPENDIX G:
Sample Program For Total Body Fitness

You can get fit in just 3 hours per week. I suggest doing aerobic exercise 3 days per week for 30 minutes and weight training 2 days per week for 45 minutes. When beginning, start with what is comfortable for your body. Being sore is not good. If you walk for 5 minutes and become fatigued - stop. Build from this point slowly (i.e. add 1 minute per walk until you reach 30 minutes. This may take a few weeks or longer, that's OK).

MON	TUE	WED	THU	FRI	SAT	SUN
Aerobics	Weights	Aerobics	OFF	Weights	Aerobics	OFF

Aerobics: To start, pick 1 or 2 activities (walk, bike, etc.). You can do one activity each aerobic exercise day or alternate from one to the other on different days (e.g. walk Monday, bike Wednesday, walk Saturday). Do not do 5 minutes of the bike, 5 minutes of treadmill, 5 minutes of stepper and 5 minutes of rower. Stick with one activity for the entire time you exercise. Remember, to get 20 minutes of aerobic benefits you need about 30 minutes of time (5 minutes for the warm-up and 5 minutes for the cool down).

Weights: Start with 1 set of 10 reps for each body part and build from there. You may want to do all exercise at home or at a gym or maybe a little at both. Just get started.

Stretching: End each workout with your stretches. Try the suggested stretches and see how they feel. You may want to make substitutions. Your routine should be comfortable.

REFERENCES

1. Southmayd, W., Rippe, J. *The Sports Performance Factors.* Putnam Publishing Group: New York, NY, 1985, p.13.
2. American College of Sports Medicine. *Guidelines for Exercise Testing and Prescription (4th Edition).* Lea and Febiger: Philadelphia, PA, 1991, p.7.
3. Stamford, B. "What is an Exercise Stress Test?" *Physician and Sports Medicine* 16(3):245-246, 1988.
4. Southmayd, W., Rippe, J. *The Sports Performance Factors.* Putnam Publishing Group: New York, NY, 1985, p.13.
5. Ibid, p.15.
6. Stamford, B. "Warming Up." *Physician and Sports Medicine* 15911):168, 1987.
7. Ibid.
8. Bailey, C. *The New Fit or Fat.* Houghton Mifflin Company: Boston, MA, 1991, p.39.
9. Ibid.
10. A Round Table, "The Health Benefits of Exercise." *Physician and Sports Medicine* 15(10):115-132, 1987.
11. American College of Sports Medicine. *Guidelines for Exercise Testing and Prescription (4th Edition).* Lea and Febiger: Philadelphia, PA, 1991, p.96.
12. Ibid, p.102.
13. American Council on Exercise. *Personal Trainer Manual.* San Diego, CA, 1991, p.202.
14. American College of Sports Medicine. *Guidelines for Exercise Testing and Prescription (4th Edition).* Lea and Febiger: Philadelphia, PA, 1991, p.96.
15. Moline, P. "The Strength Factor." *The Walking Magazine.* September/October, 1991, p.44-48.
16. Work, J. "Strength Training: A Bridge to Interdependence for the Elderly." *Physician and Sports Medicine* 17(11):134-140, 1989.
17. American Council on Exercise. *Personal Trainer Manual.* San Diego, CA, 1991, p.500.
18. Giel, D. "Women's Weight Lifting: Elevating a Sport to World Class Status." *Physician and Sports Medicine* 16(4):163-170, 1988.
19. Keleman, M., Stewart, K. "Circuit Weight Training: A New Direction for Cardiac Rehabilitation." *Sports Medicine* 2:385-388, 1985.
20. Ward, P., Ward, R. *Encyclopedia of Weight Training.* QPT Publications: Laguna Hills, CA, 1991, p.43.
21. Stamford, B. "What is Cellulite?" *Physician and Sports Medicine* 14(11):226, 1986.
22. Katch, F., McArdle, W. *Introduction to Nutrition, Exercise, and Health.* Lea & Febiger: Philadelphia, PA, 1993, p.338.
23. Stewart, K., Mason, M., Kelemen, M. "Three Year Participation in Circuit Weight Training Improves Muscular Strength and Self Efficacy in Cardiac Patients." *Journal of Cardiopulmonary Rehabilitation* 8:292-296, 1988.
24. Fleck, S., Kraemer, W. "Resistance Training: Physiological Responses and Adaptations (Part 2 of 4)." *Physician and Sport Medicine* 16(4):108-122, 1988.
25. Work, J. "Strength Training: A Bridge to Interdependence for the Elderly." *Physician and Sports Medicine* 17(11):134-140, 1989.
26. Clark, E. *Growing Old is Not for Sissies.* Pomegranate Calendars and Books: Pateluma, CA, 1986.
27. Stone, M., O'Bryant, H. *Weight Training: A Scientific Approach.* Burgess International Group, Ins.: Minneapolis, MN, 1984, p.142.
28. Ibid, pp.123-126.

29. Ward, P., Ward, R. *Encyclopedia of Weight Training*, QPT Publications: Laguna Hills, CA, 1991, p.73.

30. Keleman, M., Stewart, K. "Circuit Weight Training: A New Direction for Cardiac Rehabilitation." *Sports Medicine* 2:385-388, 1985.

31. Harman, E., Rosenstein, R., Frykman, P., Nigro, G. "Effects of a Belt on Intra-Abdominal Pressure During Weightlifting." *Medicine and Science in Sports and Exercise* 21(2):186, 1989.

32. Anderson, B. *Stretching.* Shelter Publications, Inc.: Bolinas, CA, 1980, p.9.

33. American Academy of Orthopaedic Surgery. *Athletic Training and Sports Medicine.* Park Ridge, IL, year, p.210.

34. Smith, L. "Causes of Delayed Onset Muscle Soreness and the Impact on Athletic Performance: A Review." *Journal of Applied Sport Science Research* 6(3):135-141, 1992.

35. Stone, M., Keith, R., Learney, J., Fleck, S., Wilson, G., Triplett, N. "Overtraining: A Review of the Signs, Symptoms and Possible Causes." *Journal of Applied Sport Science Research* 5(1):35-50, 1992.

36. Bailey, C. *The New Fit or Fat.* Houghton Mifflin Company: Boston, 1991, pp.9-10.

37. Ibid, p.29.

38. McArdle, W., Katch, F., Katch, V. *Exercise Physiology: Exercise, Nutrition and Human Performance.* Lea & Febiger: Malvern, PA, 1991, p.680.

39. Ibid, p.678.

40. Mahan, L., Arlin, M. *Krause's Food, Nutrition & Diet Therapy.* W.B. Saunders Company: Philadelphia, PA, 1991, pp.322-323.

41. Peterson, M., Peterson, K. *Eat to Compete: A Guide to Sports Nutrition.* Year Book Medical Publishers, Inc.,: Chicago, IL, 1988, p.157.

42. Ward, P., Ward, R. *Encyclopedia of Weight Training.* QPT Publications: Laguna Hills, CA, 1991, p.22.

43. American Council on Exercise. *Personal Trainer Manual.* San Diego, CA, 1991, p.114.

44. Ward, P., Ward, R. *Encyclopedia of Weight Training.* QPT Publications: Laguna Hills, CA, 1991, p.6.

45. Peterson, M., Peterson, K. *Eat to Compete: A Guide to Sports Nutrition.* Year Book Medical Publishers, Inc.: Chicago, IL, 1988, pp.24-31.

46. Ward, P., Ward, R. *Encyclopedia of Weight Training.* QPT Publications: Laguna Hills, CA, 1991, p.7.

47. Ward, P., Ward, R. *Encyclopedia of Weight Training.* QPT Publications: Laguna Hills, CA, 1991, pp.8-9.

48. Guthrie, H. *Introductory Nutrition.* Times Mirror/Mosby College Publishing: St. Louis, MO, 1989, p.129.

49. Ward, P., Ward, R. *Encyclopedia of Weight Training.* QPT Publications: Laguna Hills, CA, 1991, p.9-13.

50. Food and Drug Administration. "The New Food Label." *FDA Backgrounder,* 1993.

51. Ibid.

52. Ibid.

53. Ibid.

54. Ibid

55. Serfass, R. "Nutrition for the Athlete Update." *Contemporary Nutrition* 7(4), 1982.

56. Southmayd, S., Hoffman, M. *Sports Health: The Complete Book of Athletic Injuries.* The Putnam Publishing Group: New York, NY, 1981, pp.411-412.

57. Ibid.